MUSCLE MATTERS

A Nutritional Guide to Lifelong Strength

Patrick Bugeja

Book title: Muscle Matters: A Nutritional Guide to Lifelong Strength
Author: Patrick Bugeja
First edition: 2026
ISBN: 978-1-7637005-1-2
Publisher / Imprint: Active8 Publishing

Medical and Nutrition Disclaimer

This book has been written for educational purposes. It is designed to help readers better understand the relationship between skeletal muscle, nutrition, ageing, training, recovery, and long-term physical independence.

The information provided is general in nature and should not be taken as personal medical, nutritional, or exercise advice. Every person has a different health history, physical capacity, medication profile, injury background, and nutritional requirement. What is appropriate for one person may not be appropriate for another.

Before making major changes to your diet, protein intake, supplement use, resistance training, physical activity, or recovery routine, you should consult a suitably qualified health professional. This is especially important if you have a chronic health condition, kidney disease, diabetes, cardiovascular disease, osteoporosis, inflammatory disease, cancer, significant pain, recent surgery, unexplained weight loss, or any condition affecting your ability to exercise safely.

The author has made every reasonable effort to present information that is accurate and evidence-informed at the time of writing. However, health science continues to evolve, and new findings may refine or change current understanding. Readers are encouraged to use this book as a foundation for informed discussion with qualified professionals rather than as a substitute for individual assessment.

Dedication

To everyone who wants to age with strength, independence, and dignity.

And to those who refuse to accept that weakness, decline, and loss of confidence must be an unavoidable part of getting older.

Acknowledgements

This book was shaped by a simple but important belief: muscle health matters far more than most people realise.

I would like to acknowledge the researchers, clinicians, educators, and health professionals whose work continues to deepen our understanding of skeletal muscle, ageing, nutrition, exercise, and human resilience. Their contribution has made it possible to translate complex science into practical knowledge that can help people protect their strength across life.

I also acknowledge the clients, patients, students, and everyday people whose experiences highlight the real-world importance of this topic. Muscle health is not only a scientific issue. It is a human one. It affects how people move, recover, work, care for themselves, and maintain independence.

Finally, I thank those who supported the development of this book and encouraged its completion. Writing a book requires persistence, patience, and a clear purpose. This project exists because the message is worth sharing.

Author's Note

Muscle Matters was written because muscle health is still underestimated.

Many people think about ageing only in terms of wrinkles, weight, heart health, or general fitness. Far fewer think seriously about skeletal muscle until strength begins to fade, movement becomes harder, or injury and illness take longer to recover from. Yet muscle is central to how we live. It helps us move, stabilise, lift, balance, regulate blood glucose, recover from stress, and maintain independence.

This book is not written only for athletes or people who already enjoy training. It is written for anyone who wants to understand why muscle matters across the lifespan and what can be done to protect it. The aim is to bridge the gap between science and practical action. Muscle preservation is not about chasing extremes. It is about building habits that support strength, function, and resilience over time.

As a myotherapist, I have seen how much physical capacity influences quality of life. Pain, weakness, poor recovery, inactivity, and loss of confidence can gradually narrow a person's world. On the other hand, strength and movement can restore confidence, improve function, and help people stay active in their own lives for longer.

This book focuses strongly on nutrition because diet is one of the most powerful tools available for supporting muscle health. But nutrition does not work alone. Protein, resistance training, recovery, sleep, stress, inflammation, gut health, and chronic disease all interact. The body is a system, and muscle preservation works best when these parts are understood together.

My goal is not to overwhelm the reader with complicated rules. My goal is to make the science clear enough that it becomes useful. If this book helps you take muscle health more seriously, ask better questions, train more consistently, eat more intentionally, or protect your independence with greater confidence, then it has served its purpose.

How to Use This Book

This book is designed to be read in order, but it can also be returned to section by section as a reference.

The early chapters build the foundation. They explain what skeletal muscle is, how it works, how it changes with age, and why muscle loss affects far more than appearance. These chapters provide the scientific base for understanding why later strategies matter.

The middle chapters move into nutrition, protein, resistance training, recovery, dietary patterns, gut health, and the biological systems that influence muscle preservation. These sections are intended to help you understand not only what to do, but why it matters.

The later chapters apply these ideas across life stages and real-world challenges. Muscle preservation does not happen in perfect conditions. People experience pain, injury, illness, stress, ageing, appetite changes, chronic disease, and interruptions to training. This book recognises those realities and aims to provide a flexible framework rather than an unrealistic ideal.

You do not need to apply everything at once. In fact, the most effective changes are often the ones that are repeatable. Start with the major levers: regular resistance training, adequate protein, daily movement, good sleep, and a diet pattern that supports recovery and metabolic health. Once those foundations are improving, the finer details become more useful.

This book is not a replacement for professional care. If you have a medical condition, pain, injury, or uncertainty about exercise or nutrition, use the information here to guide better conversations with your doctor, dietitian, exercise professional, physiotherapist, myotherapist, or other qualified health practitioner.

Most importantly, use this book as a reminder that muscle health is not a minor detail of ageing. It is one of the foundations of independence. The earlier it is protected, the better. But it is never too late to begin.

About the Author

Patrick Bugeja is a myotherapist with a strong interest in muscle health, ageing, nutrition, movement, pain, and long-term physical independence. His clinical work focuses on helping people understand the body in a practical way, combining hands-on treatment, movement assessment, corrective exercise, and education to support better function.

Through his work in myotherapy, Patrick has seen how strength, mobility, recovery, and confidence can shape a person's quality of life. He has also seen how easily muscle health can be overlooked until weakness, pain, injury, or reduced independence begins to interfere with everyday living.

Muscle Matters: A Nutritional Guide to Lifelong Strength was written to make the science of muscle preservation clear, practical, and relevant. The book brings together evidence-informed principles from nutrition, exercise physiology, ageing biology, recovery, and clinical practice to help readers understand how muscle can be protected across the lifespan.

Patrick's goal is to help people move away from passive ideas about ageing and toward a more active understanding of physical resilience. Ageing cannot be stopped, but strength, function, and independence can often be protected far more than many people realise.

Patrick is based in Victoria, Australia.

Contents

Chapter 1: Foundations of Muscle Health and Lifelong Strength

Introduction

In the pursuit of longevity and sustained quality of life, few systems are as fundamental as the musculoskeletal system. Composed of skeletal muscle, bone, tendons, ligaments, and connective tissue, it provides both structural integrity and the capacity for movement, stability, and functional independence. It is the system that allows us to stand against gravity, coordinate complex movement, generate force, and interact physically with the world. From walking and lifting to maintaining posture and balance, everyday life depends on its ongoing performance.

Across the lifespan, this system changes. Skeletal muscle in particular is highly responsive to both use and disuse, and it becomes increasingly vulnerable to age-related decline. From as early as midlife, gradual reductions in muscle mass and strength can begin, often accelerating in later decades if not actively countered. This process—commonly referred to as sarcopenia—includes loss of muscle tissue, reduced force production, and diminished functional capacity. Early on, the changes can be easy to miss. Over time, however, they can erode mobility, balance, and resilience, increasing the risk of falls, fractures, and loss of independence.

Muscle is also far more than a mechanical engine for movement. It functions as a metabolically active organ with wide systemic influence. Skeletal muscle is a major site of glucose disposal and plays a central role in insulin sensitivity. It serves as a reservoir of amino acids used for tissue repair and recovery during illness or injury. It also releases signalling molecules that influence inflammation, vascular function, and broader physiological stability. In this sense, muscle health is not merely about strength—it is closely tied to overall health and the body's capacity to cope with stressors.

Despite its importance, muscle health is often overlooked until weakness, fatigue, or injury becomes obvious. By that point, meaningful decline may already be established, making restoration more challenging. A long-standing assumption that deterioration is an unavoidable consequence of ageing has contributed to a passive approach to prevention. Yet contemporary research consistently shows that while ageing cannot be stopped, muscle decline can often be slowed, stabilised, and in many cases improved. With appropriate resistance training, adequate dietary protein intake, and supportive lifestyle practices, muscle mass and strength can be preserved well into later life.

Muscle Matters: A Nutritional Guide to Lifelong Strength is designed to bridge the gap between scientific understanding and practical action. It provides a structured exploration of musculoskeletal physiology, the mechanisms underlying muscle ageing, and the nutritional strategies that support preservation and performance. The goal is not simply to add years to life, but to enhance healthspan—to increase the likelihood that added years are lived with strength, independence, and functional capacity.

Whether you are aiming to protect independence later in life or build habits that prevent steep decline later on, the principles in this book are grounded in physiology and supported by evidence. Muscle health is not a niche topic reserved for athletes.

It is a foundational determinant of long-term vitality, and it is one of the most modifiable aspects of ageing when approached systematically.

The Importance of Musculoskeletal Health

The musculoskeletal system is not a passive framework. It is a living, adaptive network responsible for movement, structural support, organ protection, and physical autonomy. At its centre lies skeletal muscle, which accounts for roughly 35–40 percent of total body mass in healthy adults. That tissue is not merely responsible for producing force; it influences health through mechanical, metabolic, and protective roles that become increasingly important with age.

Movement begins at the microscopic level. Within muscle fibres, highly organised structures contain the contractile proteins actin and myosin, which interact in a coordinated sliding mechanism to convert chemical energy into mechanical force. This process scales upward—across millions of fibres—allowing both fine motor control and high-force output. The ability to vary force and timing is what enables efficient movement, stable posture, balance reactions, and the capacity to tolerate physical stress.

The significance of muscle extends beyond locomotion. Skeletal muscle is the primary site of insulin-mediated glucose uptake and a cornerstone of metabolic regulation. During physical activity, muscle contraction increases glucose transport through both insulin-dependent and insulin-independent pathways, supporting blood glucose control and reducing metabolic strain. This is one reason muscle preservation is closely tied to lower risk of insulin resistance and type 2 diabetes as we age.

Muscle also serves as the body's largest reservoir of amino acids. These amino acids are not only used to build muscle itself; they are required for immune function, enzyme production, and tissue repair. During illness, injury, or periods of inadequate intake, the body may draw on muscle-derived amino acids to support critical functions. Adequate muscle mass therefore functions as a metabolic buffer, improving resilience during periods of higher physiological demand.

Because muscle is metabolically active, it contributes meaningfully to resting energy expenditure. Higher lean mass tends to support a higher resting metabolic rate, which can help with long-term body weight regulation. Conversely, as muscle mass declines, resting energy needs fall. If eating patterns remain unchanged, this shift can promote gradual fat gain, particularly visceral adiposity, which in turn contributes to systemic inflammation and metabolic dysfunction. Over time, this creates a feedback loop: reduced activity and reduced muscle accelerate metabolic decline, and metabolic decline further undermines muscle quality and function.

The functional consequences are often the most immediate. Sarcopenia is not defined only by muscle size loss. It also includes declines in neuromuscular efficiency and force production. As strength and power fall, daily tasks become more demanding: standing from a chair, climbing stairs, carrying loads, and recovering balance after a stumble. When these capacities erode, frailty risk rises, fall risk increases, and independence narrows.

At a public health level, muscle decline is not a minor issue. Reduced strength is associated with higher rates of hospitalisation, longer recovery times, greater healthcare utilisation, and increased mortality risk. On a societal scale, widespread loss of muscle function across ageing populations increases strain on healthcare systems and caregivers. Preserving musculoskeletal health is therefore not simply about performance—it is about maintaining autonomy and reducing disease burden.

The most important point is that decline is modifiable. Evidence from exercise physiology and nutrition science supports the ability of resistance training, adequate protein intake, and supportive lifestyle practices to preserve strength across the lifespan. Even in advanced age, skeletal muscle retains a remarkable capacity to adapt when appropriately challenged and nourished. Muscle preservation is not a luxury goal; it is a practical strategy for long-term health and independence.

The Role of Diet in Healthy Ageing

Physical activity is essential for maintaining strength and function, but training does not work in a vacuum. Exercise provides the stimulus that tells the body muscle is needed. Nutrition supplies the substrates and the internal environment that allow the body to respond. Without adequate energy and nutrients, the ability to repair tissue, build muscle proteins, and adapt to training is limited—especially as we age.

Protein sits at the centre of nutrition for muscle because it provides the amino acids required to maintain and rebuild lean tissue. Certain amino acids also act as signals that activate pathways involved in muscle protein synthesis after meals and after resistance training. This matters because muscle is continuously remodelled. Proteins are broken down and rebuilt every day, and the long-term outcome depends on whether that cycle tilts toward preservation often enough to maintain function across time.

With ageing, the conversation becomes more nuanced. Muscle often responds less robustly to both dietary protein and training stimuli, a phenomenon commonly described as anabolic resistance. In practical terms, it means older adults often need a stronger protein signal than younger adults to stimulate the same level of muscle protein synthesis. That does not require extremes, but it does require intention—particularly when the goal is preserving independence rather than simply avoiding deficiency.

Meal structure also matters. It is not only the total daily amount of protein, but how that protein is distributed across the day. Research suggests that spreading protein intake more evenly can support repeated stimulation of muscle protein synthesis compared with patterns that concentrate most protein into one large evening meal. This does not require perfection. It simply highlights that common modern patterns—very low protein at breakfast, moderate at lunch, high at dinner—may be less supportive of muscle preservation over decades, particularly in older adults.

Muscle health is not built on protein alone. Vitamins and minerals support the machinery that makes muscle contraction, energy production, and recovery possible. Vitamin D has well-established links to musculoskeletal function and neuromuscular performance. B vitamins support energy metabolism and tissue processes relevant to training and recovery. Ageing can also reduce nutrient absorption and endogenous production, which is one reason nutritional strategy often needs to become more deliberate over time.

Dietary fats matter as well, particularly omega-3 fatty acids, which have been studied for their influence on inflammation and anabolic signalling in certain contexts. The larger point is not that one nutrient solves the problem, but that healthy ageing is supported by nutritional alignment: adequate protein, sufficient energy, a diet quality that supports recovery, and micronutrient sufficiency that prevents hidden constraints on function.

In the chapters ahead, these principles will be explored in greater depth, with practical application grounded in physiology. The aim is to make nutrition a predictable support system for strength rather than an afterthought or a trend-driven experiment.

Integration: Beyond Isolated Interventions

Muscle preservation is rarely determined by a single habit. It reflects the interaction between mechanical stimulus, nutritional adequacy, and the body's capacity to recover and adapt. Training provides the signal. Nutrition provides the resources. Recovery determines whether those signals translate into long-term improvement or chronic fatigue and inconsistency.

A coordinated strategy therefore matters. People often approach health as separate projects—exercise on one day, diet on another, and recovery only when something breaks down. In reality, these inputs overlap. When they align, muscle adapts and function improves. When they are consistently misaligned, progress slows and decline accelerates. This book is built around that integrated reality: not as a collection of isolated interventions, but as a system for preserving strength across decades.

Why This Book Matters

Human lifespan has increased dramatically over the past century. Advances in medicine, sanitation, nutrition, and public health have reduced mortality and extended life expectancy across much of the world. Yet longer life does not automatically mean healthier life. The defining question of modern ageing is no longer only how long we live, but how well we live during those added years.

Muscle health sits at the centre of that question. Loss of muscle mass and strength is one of the most consistent predictors of frailty, loss of independence, hospitalisation, and all-cause mortality in ageing populations. Declines in muscle function are closely associated with impaired metabolic control, increased fall risk, reduced mobility, and lower quality of life. Importantly, these changes often begin decades before visible disability appears. By the time weakness becomes clinically apparent, significant decline may already be present.

Despite this, muscle health remains underemphasised in mainstream health conversations. Public attention frequently centres on cardiovascular disease, weight management, or bone density, while skeletal muscle—an organ system that influences all of these domains—receives comparatively little focus. This gap in awareness contributes to passive acceptance of muscle decline as inevitable rather than modifiable.

This book exists to challenge that assumption. The scientific literature across exercise physiology, nutrition science, and ageing biology supports a clear message: muscle mass, strength, and functional capacity remain responsive to intervention across the lifespan. Resistance training improves neuromuscular function. Nutrition—particularly adequate protein—supports repair and adaptation. When these strategies are sustained, the outcomes extend beyond strength alone into metabolic health, resilience, and independence.

The relevance is not confined to a single demographic. In early adulthood, building and maintaining muscle helps establish metabolic and structural reserve. In midlife, preserving muscle supports metabolic stability, injury resilience, and long-term function. In later life, strength and power become central to independence, fall prevention, and recovery capacity. At every stage, muscle intersects with broader health outcomes.

This book is designed as a structured, evidence-informed guide that translates physiology into practical application. It is not a collection of trends or quick fixes. Its purpose is durable physical capability—strength that supports movement, autonomy, and resilience as the years progress.

Conclusion

Muscle health is not accidental, and it is not predetermined. It is shaped by cumulative decisions made consistently over time—mechanical, nutritional, and behavioural. Understanding this shifts the perspective from passive ageing to active stewardship of one's physical capacity.

This chapter has established that skeletal muscle is more than a structural component of movement. It is a metabolically active organ system central to glucose regulation, energy expenditure, structural stability, and resilience against functional decline. Its preservation influences mobility and strength, but also broader outcomes including metabolic integrity, fall risk, independence, and healthspan.

The evidence is clear: while biological changes occur across the lifespan, the trajectory of muscle mass and function remains responsive to intervention. Resistance training provides the stimulus for adaptation. Nutrition supports repair, preservation, and recovery. When these are applied consistently, ageing is more likely to be accompanied by capability rather than progressive limitation.

The chapters that follow build this foundation progressively. We move next into the anatomy and physiology of skeletal muscle—how fibres are organised, how force is generated, and how adaptation occurs at the cellular level. From there, we will examine how nutrition and training strategies can be applied across the lifespan to preserve strength and independence. Long-term capability is not the product of isolated effort, but of informed strategy sustained over time.

Chapter 2: Skeletal Muscle Anatomy and Physiology

An Introduction to Skeletal Muscle

The human body contains three primary types of muscle tissue: skeletal, smooth, and cardiac. While all muscle shares the ability to contract, each type is built for a different role. Smooth muscle lines hollow organs and blood vessels and operates involuntarily to regulate functions such as digestion, airway calibre, and vascular tone. Cardiac muscle is found only in the heart and contracts rhythmically under specialised electrical control to maintain circulation. Skeletal muscle, the focus of this chapter, is different again: it is striated, organised into highly structured fibres, and under voluntary control through the somatic nervous system.

Skeletal muscle attaches to bone through tendons. When it contracts, it generates tension that is transmitted through the tendon to move the skeleton across joints. This makes skeletal muscle the primary engine of human movement. Yet its role extends beyond locomotion. Muscle contributes to posture and joint stability through continuous low-level activation, produces heat as a by-product of metabolism, and plays a major role in metabolic regulation through glucose uptake and substrate use. Because skeletal muscle is both mechanically powerful and metabolically active, its health influences performance, resilience, and long-term function.

This chapter establishes the physiological foundation for the rest of the book. We will explore how skeletal muscle is structured, how it contracts, how fibre types differ, how the nervous system controls force, how muscle repairs and adapts, and how energy systems support muscular work.

Muscle Structure and Composition

To understand how skeletal muscle produces force, it helps to see it as a hierarchy of structures arranged with remarkable precision. A whole muscle is made of bundles, and those bundles are made of fibres, and each fibre contains the contractile machinery that produces tension. This layered architecture allows microscopic events inside a cell to scale up into whole-body movement.

At the cellular level, the basic unit is the muscle fibre. A muscle fibre is a long, cylindrical, multinucleated cell formed during development when precursor cells fuse. The presence of multiple nuclei supports the high protein turnover required for ongoing repair and adaptation. The fibre is surrounded by the sarcolemma, a specialised membrane responsible for conducting electrical signals and maintaining structural integrity. Inside the fibre, the sarcoplasm contains organelles, enzymes, energy substrates, and the contractile structures that enable repeated contraction.

Within each muscle fibre are myofibrils, long thread-like structures aligned in parallel. Myofibrils are made of repeating units called sarcomeres, which are the smallest functional units of contraction. Sarcomeres are arranged end-to-end along the myofibril, and thousands of sarcomeres shortening together produce measurable fibre shortening. Millions of sarcomeres contracting across many fibres produce whole-muscle force.

Each sarcomere contains thin filaments composed mainly of actin and thick filaments composed mainly of myosin. The actin filaments anchor to Z-discs at each end of the sarcomere, while myosin sits centrally. This arrangement creates the striated appearance of skeletal muscle. Descriptions such as I-bands, A-bands, H-zones, and the M-line refer to regions defined by filament overlap, and they reflect the mechanical structure that allows contraction to occur efficiently.

Muscle fibres are grouped into fascicles, and fascicles into a whole muscle. Surrounding and integrating these structures are connective tissue layers that support alignment, distribute force, and provide the pathway through which contractile tension reaches the tendon. The endomysium surrounds each fibre, the perimysium surrounds each fascicle, and the epimysium surrounds the entire muscle. These layers blend into the tendon, meaning that force generated at the sarcomere level is transmitted through connective tissue to bone. This is why muscle function depends not only on contractile proteins but also on the integrity and mechanical properties of connective tissue and tendon.

This structural hierarchy also explains why muscle quality matters. A muscle can appear similar in size while differing greatly in functional capacity if connective tissue stiffness, intramuscular fat, fibre size, or neuromuscular control changes. These ideas become increasingly important when we later discuss ageing and long-term preservation.

Muscle Contraction Mechanism

Skeletal muscle contraction depends on a sequence that links a neural signal to mechanical force at the sarcomere. This process is often called excitation–contraction coupling. It ensures that voluntary intent becomes coordinated action.

Contraction begins with a motor command originating in the central nervous system. The signal travels along a motor neuron and reaches the neuromuscular junction, the specialised synapse between the nerve terminal and the muscle fibre. When the nerve impulse arrives, acetylcholine is released into the synaptic cleft and binds to receptors on the sarcolemma. This triggers depolarisation of the muscle fibre. If the signal reaches threshold, an action potential is generated and spreads across the sarcolemma.

To ensure rapid activation throughout the fibre, the action potential travels down transverse tubules, invaginations of the membrane that carry the electrical signal deep into the cell. This triggers calcium release from the sarcoplasmic reticulum, the fibre's specialised calcium storage system. The rise in intracellular calcium is the key step that allows cross-bridge cycling to begin.

At rest, binding sites on actin are blocked by tropomyosin. The troponin complex regulates tropomyosin's position. When calcium binds to troponin, the complex changes shape and shifts tropomyosin away from actin's binding sites. Myosin heads can then bind to actin and generate force.

The cross-bridge cycle is powered by ATP. Myosin binds to actin, performs a power stroke that pulls actin toward the centre of the sarcomere, and then detaches when ATP binds to myosin. ATP is hydrolysed to reset the myosin head into a high energy position, allowing the cycle to repeat. As long as calcium remains elevated and ATP is available, the cycle continues and the muscle maintains tension or shortens.

Relaxation is also energy dependent. When neural stimulation stops, calcium is pumped back into the sarcoplasmic reticulum through ATP-powered pumps. As calcium levels fall, tropomyosin re-covers the binding sites, cross-bridge formation stops, and the muscle returns toward resting tension. This is why ATP is required not only for contraction but for relaxation as well.

Types of Muscle Fibres

Skeletal muscle is composed of fibre types that differ in contraction speed, force potential, fatigue resistance, and metabolic profile. These differences influence performance and help explain why ageing affects strength and power differently across the lifespan.

Type I fibres, often called slow-twitch fibres, are specialised for sustained, lower-intensity activity. They contract more slowly and produce lower peak force but resist fatigue well. Their structure supports aerobic metabolism, typically featuring higher mitochondrial density, greater capillary supply, and higher myoglobin content. These fibres are heavily involved in posture and endurance-oriented tasks.

Type II fibres, often called fast-twitch fibres, are designed for rapid, high-force contractions. They generate greater force and power but fatigue faster. They rely more on phosphocreatine and glycolytic pathways to rapidly regenerate ATP during intense effort. Type II fibres are commonly described as Type IIa and Type IIx. Type IIa fibres have both oxidative and glycolytic characteristics, making them adaptable and important for repeated high-intensity efforts. Type IIx fibres contract fastest and produce high power but fatigue quickly and are more prominent in maximal or explosive actions.

Fibre type distribution varies between individuals and between muscles, influenced by genetics, activity history, and training. While complete conversion between Type I and Type II is limited, shifts within Type II characteristics can occur with training or disuse. This adaptability is part of why resistance training can preserve or restore function even after periods of decline.

Ageing tends to affect Type II fibres disproportionately. This selective vulnerability contributes to the common pattern where power and rapid force production decline more steeply than endurance. Because power underpins balance recovery and quick stabilising responses, the preservation of Type II fibre function has strong relevance for independence in later life.

Neuromuscular Function

Muscle strength is not determined by muscle tissue alone. The nervous system governs how effectively muscle fibres are recruited, how quickly force is produced, and how precisely movement is controlled. For many people, the "feel" of strength and coordination reflects neuromuscular efficiency as much as muscle size.

The basic unit of neuromuscular control is the motor unit, consisting of a motor neuron and the muscle fibres it innervates. When the motor neuron fires, all fibres within that unit contract together. Motor units vary in size. Muscles requiring fine control tend to have small motor units for precise force modulation, while large locomotor muscles tend to have larger motor units capable of high force output.

Force is regulated by recruitment and firing rate. Recruitment generally follows the size principle: smaller, fatigue-resistant motor units are activated first, and larger, higher-threshold units are recruited as force demands increase. Force can also be increased by raising firing frequency, which allows summation of contractile responses and faster, stronger contractions.

This explains why early strength gains with resistance training often occur before visible hypertrophy. Improvements in coordination, recruitment efficiency, movement skill, and reduced unnecessary co-contraction can increase force output rapidly. Over time, training can also influence muscle size and fibre characteristics, but the nervous system remains a major driver of how strength is expressed.

Ageing affects neuromuscular function as well. Motor neuron loss reduces the total number of functioning motor units. Some denervated fibres may be reinnervated by surviving neurons, which can preserve fibres but results in fewer, larger motor units. This pattern can reduce fine control and contribute to slower, less precise movement. These changes help explain why strength and power can decline faster than muscle mass alone would predict.

Muscle Development and Repair

Skeletal muscle is dynamic tissue that adapts to repeated demand. Resistance training provides mechanical tension and metabolic stress that stimulate remodelling. Over time, muscle can increase its force-producing capacity, improve coordination, and in many cases increase fibre size.

Hypertrophy refers to an increase in fibre cross-sectional area. It is driven primarily by mechanotransduction: the conversion of mechanical loading into intracellular signals that influence gene expression and protein synthesis. Hypertrophy reflects repeated cycles where muscle protein synthesis exceeds muscle protein breakdown over time, supported by adequate recovery and nutrition.

Satellite cells, the muscle's resident stem cells, contribute to repair and adaptation. In response to overload or injury, satellite cells can activate, proliferate, and fuse with existing fibres. This can increase myonuclear number, supporting the fibre's capacity for protein synthesis and long-term maintenance. This process becomes especially relevant when discussing ageing, because regenerative capacity tends to decline, which is one reason consistent training and adequate nutrition matter more in later decades.

Nutrition supports muscle development by providing amino acids for protein synthesis. Resistance training increases muscle protein synthesis for hours after a session, and dietary protein provides the building blocks required to capitalise on that response. When intake is inadequate, the adaptive response is blunted. When training and nutrition align consistently, the body becomes more likely to preserve and improve muscle function across time.

Muscle Energy Systems and Metabolism

All muscle contraction depends on ATP, the immediate energy currency required for cross-bridge cycling and calcium handling. Because stored ATP in muscle is limited, ATP must be regenerated continuously during activity. The body uses three overlapping energy systems to do this, with their relative contribution determined by intensity and duration.

The phosphagen system provides immediate ATP resynthesis during brief, high-intensity efforts such as maximal lifting or sprinting. Phosphocreatine donates a phosphate group to ADP to rapidly regenerate ATP. This system delivers ATP at a high rate but for only a short duration because phosphocreatine stores are limited.

The glycolytic system contributes more as high-intensity activity continues. Anaerobic glycolysis breaks down glucose or glycogen to generate ATP at a moderate rate. When demand is high, pyruvate may be converted to lactate. Lactate itself is not the primary cause of fatigue. Fatigue is better understood as the result of the broader metabolic environment associated with high-rate glycolysis, including changes in acidity, ion balance, and cellular homeostasis.

The oxidative system supports longer-duration, lower-intensity activity. It generates ATP more slowly but with greater overall yield, using carbohydrates and fats in the presence of oxygen. This system depends on mitochondrial function and is strongly supported by Type I fibre characteristics such as higher mitochondrial density and capillary supply.

No physical activity relies on one system exclusively. Contribution shifts along a continuum, and all three systems interact. Resistance training and sprinting tend to develop phosphagen and glycolytic capacity, while endurance training increases mitochondrial density and oxidative efficiency. Ageing can influence metabolic capacity, but training remains a powerful tool for maintaining and improving energy system function across the lifespan.

Conclusion

This chapter provides the foundation for understanding muscle health across the lifespan. We examined the hierarchical structure of skeletal muscle and how sarcomeres generate force, how connective tissue integrates and transmits that force, and how contraction is controlled through calcium release and ATP-dependent cross-bridge cycling. We explored fibre types and how their metabolic and functional differences influence performance, adaptation, and the characteristic decline in power seen with ageing. We also examined neuromuscular control, highlighting that strength is partly a skill governed by recruitment and coordination, and we outlined the mechanisms that drive muscle repair and adaptation. Finally, we reviewed the energy systems that regenerate ATP and sustain muscular work.

With this framework established, the chapters that follow can examine how muscle changes with age and how nutrition and training strategies can preserve strength, function, and independence over time.

Chapter 3: Muscle Ageing: What Happens Over Time

Introduction to Muscle Ageing

Ageing brings visible changes—alterations in skin elasticity, hair pigmentation, and body composition—but some of the most impactful transformations occur within skeletal muscle. Beneath the surface, muscle tissue undergoes gradual structural, neural, and metabolic shifts that influence strength, endurance, coordination, and overall resilience. These changes are not abrupt; they accumulate progressively across decades.

The clinical term used to describe age-related loss of skeletal muscle mass and function is sarcopenia. Derived from the Greek words sarx (flesh) and penia (loss), sarcopenia reflects more than simple muscle shrinkage. It encompasses reductions in muscle fibre size, alterations in fibre type distribution, diminished motor unit integrity, impaired regenerative capacity, and decreased metabolic efficiency.

Research suggests that measurable declines in muscle mass can begin as early as the fourth decade of life. By the seventh and eighth decades, individuals may lose 20–40% of their peak muscle mass if no preventive strategies are implemented. Importantly, strength declines at an even faster rate than mass, largely due to neural changes and reductions in fast-twitch fibre function.

Muscle ageing is not merely a cosmetic concern. Skeletal muscle is central to glucose regulation, mobility, balance, thermoregulation, and independence. Its decline contributes to frailty, increased fall risk, metabolic dysfunction, and reduced capacity to recover from illness or injury. In many cases, muscle deterioration initiates a feedback loop: reduced strength leads to reduced activity, which accelerates further muscle loss.

Yet sarcopenia is not uniform in its progression. Genetics, physical activity, nutrition, hormonal status, inflammation, and chronic disease all influence its trajectory. Resistance training and adequate protein intake have repeatedly demonstrated the ability to preserve and even restore muscle function in older adults. This distinction is critical: while ageing is inevitable, accelerated muscle decline is not.

Understanding what changes within muscle tissue over time provides the foundation for intervention. In this chapter, we will examine the biological mechanisms underlying muscle ageing, the modifiable factors that influence its progression, and the evidence-based strategies that can preserve strength and independence throughout life.

Biological Mechanisms of Age-Related Muscle Change

Skeletal muscle does not simply diminish with age; it remodels. The process is gradual, multifactorial, and deeply interconnected. Structural alterations within the muscle fibres themselves interact with neural changes, hormonal shifts, inflammatory signalling, and metabolic adaptations. Over time, these cumulative influences reshape both the composition and the performance capacity of skeletal muscle.

Muscle mass typically peaks in early adulthood and then enters a slow, progressive decline. This reduction is not linear. It accelerates when compounded by inactivity, illness, or metabolic dysfunction. Importantly, the loss of strength consistently outpaces the loss of mass. This distinction matters. Muscle performance depends not only on tissue quantity, but on fibre quality, motor unit integrity, excitation–contraction efficiency, and metabolic support. Ageing affects each of these domains.

One of the most consistent structural findings in ageing muscle is the preferential atrophy and loss of Type II (fast-twitch) fibres. These fibres are responsible for rapid, high-force contractions and play a crucial role in power generation and balance recovery. As Type II fibres shrink or are lost entirely, overall muscle cross-sectional area declines, but more significantly, the ability to generate force quickly is compromised. The implications extend beyond athletic performance. Rapid force production is essential for preventing falls, climbing stairs, rising from a chair, or reacting to instability. When fast-twitch capacity diminishes, functional reserve narrows.

At the cellular level, age-related muscle loss reflects disruptions in protein turnover. Muscle tissue is in a constant state of renewal, balancing protein synthesis with protein breakdown. With advancing age, this equilibrium becomes less responsive to anabolic stimuli—a phenomenon often referred to as anabolic resistance. Older muscle demonstrates a blunted synthetic response to dietary protein and mechanical loading. Even when adequate amino acids are available, intracellular signalling pathways that regulate muscle protein synthesis, particularly those involving mTOR activation, become less sensitive. Over decades, this subtle inefficiency contributes to measurable tissue loss.

Muscle regeneration capacity also declines. Satellite cells—resident muscle stem cells located between the basal lamina and sarcolemma—are central to repair and adaptation. In youth, these cells activate in response to injury or overload, proliferate, and fuse with existing fibres to support growth and regeneration. With ageing, both satellite cell number and functional responsiveness decrease, especially in Type II fibres. This limits the muscle's ability to repair microdamage efficiently and reduces its adaptive potential following mechanical stress. The result is not an inability to adapt, but a requirement for more consistent stimulus and sufficient recovery to achieve similar outcomes.

Changes in muscle quality further compound these structural alterations. Ageing muscle frequently exhibits increased intramuscular adipose infiltration, a process termed myosteatosis. Fat accumulation between and within muscle fibres reduces the proportion of contractile tissue and interferes with effective force transmission. In parallel, connective tissue content often increases, contributing to stiffness and altered mechanical properties. These compositional changes may not dramatically alter gross muscle size initially, but they significantly impair force production efficiency and metabolic function.

The nervous system plays an equally critical role in muscle ageing. Motor neuron loss begins subtly and progresses with age, leading to a reduction in the total number of functioning motor units. When motor neurons degenerate, the muscle fibres they innervate become denervated. Some fibres are rescued through collateral reinnervation by neighbouring neurons, resulting in larger but fewer motor units. While this compensatory process preserves some muscle fibres, it alters recruitment patterns and reduces fine motor control. High-threshold motor units, which predominantly innervate fast-twitch fibres, are particularly vulnerable. The cumulative effect is diminished coordination, slower activation, reduced maximal firing rates, and impaired rapid force development.

Hormonal changes further influence this landscape. Ageing is associated with gradual declines in anabolic hormones such as testosterone, growth hormone, and insulin-like growth factor-1 (IGF-1). These hormones modulate muscle protein synthesis, satellite cell activation, and neuromuscular function. While hormonal decline alone does not cause sarcopenia, it lowers the anabolic environment in which muscle maintenance occurs. In parallel, increased systemic inflammation—often termed "inflammaging"—introduces chronic low-grade elevations in pro-inflammatory cytokines. These signalling molecules can accelerate protein breakdown, impair anabolic signalling, and contribute to metabolic dysregulation.

Mitochondrial function also evolves over time. Ageing muscle often demonstrates reductions in mitochondrial density and efficiency, alongside increased oxidative stress. Reactive oxygen species accumulate, and antioxidant defences may become less robust. Although oxidative stress is a normal by-product of metabolism, excessive accumulation damages cellular structures, including proteins and mitochondrial DNA. Impaired mitochondrial function reduces ATP availability and endurance capacity, further limiting overall performance and recovery potential.

These mechanisms do not operate independently. Neural decline amplifies fibre atrophy. Hormonal shifts interact with anabolic resistance. Inflammation affects mitochondrial efficiency and regenerative capacity. Physical inactivity accelerates each pathway. Muscle ageing, therefore, is not the result of a single defect but the convergence of multiple, interacting biological processes unfolding gradually across the lifespan.

Understanding these mechanisms clarifies why muscle function declines in both strength and power, why recovery becomes slower, and why metabolic resilience weakens with age. More importantly, it highlights that the ageing muscle remains biologically active and responsive—though its responsiveness requires more deliberate support. The processes described here are progressive, but they are also modifiable to varying degrees, a distinction that will guide the discussion of contributing factors and evidence-based strategies in the sections that follow.

Contributing Factors That Accelerate Muscle Ageing

While the biological processes underlying muscle ageing unfold gradually across the lifespan, their trajectory is not fixed. Intrinsic mechanisms create vulnerability, but external influences determine the speed and severity of decline. In many individuals, the most significant driver of accelerated muscle loss is not chronological age itself, but the cumulative effect of modifiable lifestyle and health factors.

Physical inactivity sits at the centre of this acceleration. Skeletal muscle is metabolically expensive tissue. It requires regular mechanical loading to justify its maintenance. When activity levels fall, protein synthesis decreases, neuromuscular recruitment becomes less efficient, and Type II fibres atrophy more rapidly. Even short periods of disuse—such as bed rest, immobilisation, or illness—can produce measurable losses in muscle mass and strength, particularly in older adults. Recovery from these periods is often incomplete, especially when repeated episodes occur over time. A sedentary lifestyle therefore compounds the intrinsic vulnerabilities already present in ageing muscle.

Nutritional inadequacy further amplifies decline. Adequate dietary protein is essential to stimulate muscle protein synthesis, yet total protein intake often decreases with age due to reduced appetite, altered taste perception, dental issues, financial constraints, or convenience-driven food choices. Beyond quantity, distribution matters. Large gaps between protein-containing meals limit repeated stimulation of muscle protein synthesis, and low-quality protein sources may provide insufficient essential amino acids—particularly leucine, a key regulator of anabolic signalling. Chronic underconsumption creates a persistent negative protein balance that gradually erodes lean tissue.

Energy deficiency also plays a role. In attempts to lose weight or manage metabolic conditions, some individuals adopt prolonged caloric restriction without resistance training or adequate protein intake. While fat loss may occur, muscle mass is often lost concurrently. Repeated cycles of weight loss and regain, particularly without structured strength training, can progressively reduce lean mass over time.

Hormonal changes interact with these behavioural factors. Gradual declines in testosterone, oestrogen, growth hormone, and insulin-like growth factor-1 reduce the anabolic environment necessary for muscle maintenance. In men, lower testosterone levels are associated with reduced muscle mass and strength. In women, the menopausal transition introduces shifts in body composition, including increased fat mass and reduced lean tissue. While hormonal decline alone does not determine muscle loss, when combined with inactivity and inadequate nutrition, it accelerates it.

Chronic low-grade inflammation represents another compounding factor. Conditions such as obesity, type 2 diabetes, cardiovascular disease, and autoimmune disorders are associated with elevated circulating inflammatory markers. These cytokines promote protein breakdown pathways and interfere with anabolic signalling. Over time, this inflammatory milieu contributes to muscle catabolism and impairs recovery from physical stressors. Adipose tissue itself acts as an endocrine organ, producing inflammatory mediators that further exacerbate muscle decline when excess fat mass accumulates.

Metabolic dysfunction adds another layer of complexity. Insulin resistance reduces the muscle's capacity to uptake glucose efficiently and impairs its anabolic response to feeding. Because skeletal muscle is the primary site of glucose disposal, reductions in muscle mass worsen glycaemic control, creating a reciprocal cycle in which metabolic disease and muscle loss reinforce one another.

Sleep disturbances, often underappreciated, also influence muscle health. Inadequate or fragmented sleep disrupts growth hormone secretion, elevates cortisol, and alters glucose metabolism. Over time, poor sleep quality can impair recovery, blunt training adaptations, and contribute to both muscle loss and fat gain.

Psychological stress similarly affects the muscle environment. Chronic elevation of cortisol promotes protein breakdown and reduces protein synthesis. While acute stress responses are adaptive, persistent activation of stress pathways shifts the balance toward catabolism. When stress coexists with poor sleep, inadequate nutrition, and inactivity, its impact is magnified.

Medication use must also be acknowledged. Long-term corticosteroid therapy, certain chemotherapeutic agents, and prolonged statin intolerance in susceptible individuals can negatively influence muscle integrity. These effects vary widely depending on dosage, duration, and individual susceptibility, but they illustrate that muscle ageing does not occur in isolation from broader medical management.

Importantly, these accelerating factors rarely occur alone. Physical inactivity often coexists with metabolic dysfunction. Poor sleep frequently accompanies chronic stress. Inadequate protein intake may coincide with caloric restriction or illness. The convergence of these influences explains why muscle ageing progresses rapidly in some individuals while remaining relatively stable in others of similar chronological age.

The key insight is this: chronological ageing creates biological susceptibility, but environmental exposure determines expression. When muscle is underloaded, undernourished, inflamed, metabolically impaired, or hormonally unsupported, decline accelerates. When these pressures are mitigated, progression slows considerably.

Recognising these contributors is essential before discussing intervention. Without understanding what drives acceleration, strategies to preserve muscle health remain incomplete. The following section will examine the functional consequences that emerge when these factors remain unaddressed.

Functional Consequences of Muscle Loss

The gradual loss of muscle mass and strength is not merely a laboratory finding or a diagnostic category; it is a functional event with tangible consequences. As skeletal muscle declines in size, quality, and neuromuscular efficiency, the effects begin to surface in everyday tasks long before clinical thresholds are reached.

One of the earliest and most significant changes is reduced strength relative to body weight. When maximal force production decreases, movements that were once automatic begin to demand greater effort. Rising from a chair, climbing stairs, carrying groceries, or maintaining posture for prolonged periods require a higher percentage of available capacity. This narrowing of functional reserve is subtle at first. Over time, however, it reduces margin for error. Tasks that once required 30 percent of maximal strength may require 50 percent or more. Fatigue accumulates more quickly, and endurance diminishes.

Loss of power is even more consequential than loss of strength. Power reflects the ability to generate force rapidly, and it declines earlier and more sharply than maximal force alone. Because many protective responses depend on speed—stepping quickly to prevent a fall, stabilising the trunk during perturbation, or catching oneself during a misstep—reduced power significantly increases fall risk. In older adults, impaired rapid force production is strongly associated with mobility limitations and loss of independence.

Balance and coordination also deteriorate as motor unit remodelling progresses. Fewer motor units, altered recruitment patterns, and slower neural firing rates reduce fine motor control. Movements become less precise and more energetically costly. Gait speed often slows. Variability in step length and stride timing increases. These subtle changes precede overt instability and serve as early markers of neuromuscular ageing.

Metabolic consequences unfold alongside functional ones. Skeletal muscle is the largest site of glucose disposal in the body. When muscle mass decreases, glucose regulation becomes less efficient. Insulin sensitivity declines, and postprandial glucose excursions become more pronounced. Over time, this contributes to increased risk of type 2 diabetes and metabolic syndrome. Reduced muscle mass also lowers resting metabolic rate, making weight maintenance more challenging and increasing the likelihood of fat accumulation, particularly visceral adiposity.

The interaction between muscle loss and bone health further compounds risk. Reduced mechanical loading on bone accelerates bone mineral density decline. Simultaneously, diminished muscle strength increases fall probability. The combination of weaker bones and higher fall risk markedly elevates fracture incidence in older adults. Recovery from fracture is often prolonged, and extended periods of immobilisation can trigger further muscle loss, creating a cycle of decline.

Hospitalisation illustrates this vulnerability clearly. Periods of acute illness frequently involve bed rest or markedly reduced mobility. Older individuals can lose significant muscle mass within days of inactivity. Recovery following discharge may be incomplete, especially if structured rehabilitation and nutritional support are absent. Each hospital episode therefore carries the potential to shift baseline function downward.

Beyond physical performance, muscle loss influences resilience. Individuals with greater muscle mass and strength demonstrate improved recovery from illness, better tolerance to surgical stress, and reduced mortality risk in a range of chronic conditions. Muscle functions not only as a mechanical tissue but as an endocrine organ, releasing myokines that influence inflammation, metabolic regulation, and systemic health. As muscle tissue declines, these protective effects diminish.

Importantly, the consequences of muscle loss are not binary. They exist on a continuum. Early reductions in strength or power may not be perceived as problematic, yet they represent progressive narrowing of physiological reserve. When reserve becomes critically low, minor stressors—an infection, a fall, a short period of inactivity—can precipitate disproportionate functional decline.

The significance of these outcomes reframes muscle ageing. It is not simply about aesthetics or athletic performance; it is about autonomy. The capacity to move independently, maintain balance, regulate metabolism, recover from stress, and preserve quality of life is deeply tied to skeletal muscle integrity. Understanding these consequences clarifies why prevention and preservation are not optional considerations but central pillars of healthy ageing.

Evidence-Based Strategies to Mitigate Muscle Ageing

Although muscle ageing is biologically programmed to some degree, its progression is highly modifiable. Skeletal muscle remains remarkably responsive to appropriate stimulus across the lifespan. The difference between inevitable ageing and accelerated decline lies largely in whether the tissue continues to receive mechanical, nutritional, and metabolic signals sufficient to justify its preservation.

Resistance training is the most robust and consistently supported intervention for mitigating age-related muscle loss. Mechanical loading stimulates muscle protein synthesis, enhances neuromuscular recruitment, and promotes hypertrophy, particularly in Type II fibres that are most vulnerable to ageing. Contrary to outdated assumptions, older adults retain the capacity to increase muscle mass and strength significantly when exposed to structured progressive resistance training. Improvements are observed not only in cross-sectional area but also in motor unit activation efficiency and rate of force development.

Importantly, the stimulus must be progressive. Muscle adapts only when challenged beyond habitual demand. Training intensity, volume, and frequency must be sufficient to activate high-threshold motor units while allowing adequate recovery. Research consistently supports resistance training performed two to three times per week, targeting major muscle groups with moderate to high intensity relative to individual capacity. Even individuals in advanced age demonstrate measurable improvements when appropriately supervised and progressed.

Nutrition acts synergistically with mechanical loading. Adequate dietary protein intake is essential to stimulate muscle protein synthesis, particularly in the context of anabolic resistance. Older adults often require a higher relative protein intake compared to younger individuals to achieve the same anabolic response. High-quality protein sources rich in essential amino acids—especially leucine—play a central role in activating intracellular signalling pathways responsible for muscle repair and growth.

Equally important is protein distribution. Spreading protein intake evenly across meals appears to stimulate repeated elevations in muscle protein synthesis throughout the day, rather than concentrating intake in a single large meal. Combining protein ingestion with resistance exercise further amplifies the anabolic response, as mechanical loading sensitises muscle tissue to amino acid availability.

Total energy balance must also be considered. Chronic caloric deficit without resistance training accelerates lean mass loss. When fat reduction is required for metabolic health, preserving muscle demands sufficient protein intake and continued mechanical loading. Intentional weight loss in older adults should therefore prioritise lean mass retention, not simply scale reduction.

Vitamin D status influences muscle function and fall risk. Deficiency is associated with impaired muscle strength and increased incidence of falls, particularly in older populations. While supplementation is not universally required, maintaining adequate vitamin D levels supports neuromuscular function and skeletal integrity.

Emerging evidence also supports the potential role of omega-3 fatty acids in enhancing muscle protein synthesis and reducing inflammation. While not a substitute for resistance training or protein intake, adequate omega-3 consumption may improve anabolic sensitivity in ageing muscle.

Beyond structured exercise and nutrition, daily movement matters. Non-exercise physical activity—walking, stair climbing, gardening, and general mobility—provides consistent low-level mechanical signalling that supports metabolic health and reduces prolonged sedentary exposure. Extended inactivity suppresses muscle protein synthesis and impairs glucose regulation even in otherwise healthy individuals. Interrupting sedentary time may therefore contribute meaningfully to muscle preservation.

Sleep and recovery are equally foundational. Growth hormone secretion, tissue repair, and neuromuscular recovery processes are closely tied to sleep quality. Chronic sleep deprivation elevates cortisol, impairs glucose metabolism, and blunts adaptive responses to training. Ensuring sufficient restorative sleep supports the biological environment required for muscle maintenance.

Management of chronic disease also influences outcomes. Optimising glycaemic control, reducing systemic inflammation, and addressing hormonal imbalances where clinically appropriate can attenuate secondary drivers of muscle loss. While pharmacological interventions are not primary prevention strategies for sarcopenia, comprehensive medical management enhances the effectiveness of lifestyle-based approaches.

The most important principle emerging from the literature is consistency. Muscle preservation is not achieved through sporadic effort but through sustained mechanical and nutritional signalling over time. Even modest but regular resistance training combined with adequate protein intake produces meaningful protection against decline. Conversely, intermittent periods of activity separated by prolonged inactivity yield limited long-term benefit.

Crucially, muscle tissue remains plastic. Even after significant loss, improvements are possible. While peak youthful capacity may not be fully restored, functional independence, strength, and metabolic resilience can be substantially enhanced at virtually any age. The biological systems governing adaptation persist; they simply require sufficient stimulus.

Mitigating muscle ageing, therefore, is not about preventing time from passing. It is about ensuring that skeletal muscle continues to receive the signals necessary to justify its maintenance. When mechanical loading, adequate nutrition, metabolic health, and recovery are aligned, muscle remains responsive. When these signals are absent, decline accelerates.

This understanding reframes ageing not as an unavoidable descent, but as a process strongly shaped by behaviour and environment.

Conclusion

Muscle ageing is neither abrupt nor arbitrary. It is the cumulative expression of structural remodelling, neural reorganisation, metabolic adaptation, hormonal change, and environmental influence unfolding over decades. The decline in muscle mass and function that characterises later life does not arise from a single defect, but from the gradual interaction of biological susceptibility and behavioural exposure.

Throughout this chapter, we have examined how skeletal muscle changes at the cellular and systemic levels, why strength declines faster than mass, and how preferential loss of fast-twitch fibres, motor unit remodelling, anabolic resistance, inflammation, and mitochondrial inefficiency collectively shape the ageing phenotype. We have also explored the compounding factors that accelerate this process—physical inactivity, inadequate protein intake, metabolic dysfunction, chronic stress, sleep disturbance, and systemic inflammation—alongside the functional consequences that follow when muscle integrity is not preserved.

The implications extend well beyond strength alone. Muscle health influences mobility, balance, metabolic regulation, resilience to illness, fracture risk, recovery capacity, and independence. It functions as both a mechanical and metabolic organ, central to the maintenance of autonomy across the lifespan. When muscle reserve narrows, vulnerability increases. When reserve is maintained, adaptability persists.

Perhaps the most important insight is this: while ageing is inevitable, accelerated muscle decline is not. Skeletal muscle remains responsive to mechanical loading and adequate nutrition throughout life. Even in advanced age, meaningful improvements in strength, coordination, and metabolic health are achievable when stimulus and recovery are appropriately aligned. The biological systems that govern adaptation do not disappear with age; they simply require deliberate support.

Understanding muscle ageing reframes the broader discussion of nutrition and training. Preserving muscle is not about aesthetics or performance optimisation alone. It is about maintaining physiological reserve, protecting independence, and sustaining quality of life. The decisions made in midlife—and earlier—compound over time, shaping the trajectory of later decades.

With the mechanisms of muscle ageing clarified, the remainder of this book will turn increasingly toward application. Nutrition, recovery, supplementation, and training strategies will be explored in greater depth, not as isolated interventions, but as coordinated tools designed to support lifelong strength.

Muscle matters because it underpins movement, metabolism, and resilience. Protecting it is not optional; it is foundational to ageing well.

Chapter 4: The Science of Nutrition and Muscle Health

Introduction

Muscle is not maintained by exercise alone. Training provides the mechanical stimulus, but nutrition determines whether that stimulus is translated into repair, adaptation, and long-term preservation—or whether muscle gradually loses ground over time. This is not just a matter of "fuel." Nutrient intake shapes the internal biochemical environment that governs how skeletal muscle behaves day to day.

At the centre of muscle regulation is a constant turnover of tissue. Proteins within skeletal muscle are continuously being broken down and rebuilt. Whether muscle is preserved, gained, or lost depends on the ongoing balance between muscle protein synthesis and muscle protein breakdown. Feeding and exercise shift that balance toward synthesis, while fasting, illness, and inadequate intake tend to favour breakdown. Nutritional intake, especially dietary protein and essential amino acids, is therefore one of the main levers controlling muscle maintenance across the lifespan.

This becomes increasingly important with age. Older muscle does not respond to nutrition and training signals as efficiently as younger muscle. The term often used to describe this reduced responsiveness is anabolic resistance—a blunted stimulation of muscle protein synthesis after protein ingestion and, in many cases, after exercise. The practical implication is straightforward: when dietary intake is marginal, older adults are more likely to sit in a net negative protein balance across weeks and months, even if calorie intake seems "adequate." Over time, that quiet imbalance contributes to measurable losses in muscle mass and function.

Nutrition, then, is not simply supportive. It is regulatory. It influences whether muscle adapts effectively to training, whether it recovers efficiently from daily loading, and whether age-related decline is slowed or accelerated. In the sections that follow, we will examine the evidence for how protein intake regulates muscle protein synthesis, how protein amount and distribution shape anabolic signalling, and how these principles shift across the lifespan.

Protein and the Regulation of Muscle Protein Synthesis

If there is one nutritional factor that consistently shows up as central to muscle health, it is protein intake. Protein provides amino acids—the raw materials required to repair damaged proteins, rebuild contractile structures, and support the ongoing remodelling that keeps muscle functional. But protein is not only structural. It is also signalling. The availability of essential amino acids directly influences the activation of pathways involved in muscle protein synthesis, shaping whether the body moves toward maintenance, growth, or loss over time.

A key concept here is that muscle does not respond equally to all protein exposures. The stimulus depends on both quantity and composition. Essential amino acids drive the synthesis response, and leucine is often discussed as a particularly influential trigger within the broader essential amino acid profile. The "leucine trigger" hypothesis proposes that reaching a threshold of leucine availability plays a key role in initiating anabolic signalling. That said, the evidence base also emphasises that this is not a leucine-only story: total essential amino acid availability, overall protein dose, and the surrounding physiological context all influence whether synthesis meaningfully increases.

Ageing shifts this responsiveness. The evidence summarised in anabolic resistance research supports the idea that older adults typically require a stronger protein stimulus to achieve the same rise in muscle protein synthesis seen in younger individuals. This is one of the reasons why evidence-based protein recommendations for older adults often exceed the minimum adult baseline. In other words, the question becomes less about "meeting the minimum" and more about meeting the dose needed to produce a meaningful anabolic signal in ageing muscle.

This is where consensus recommendations become useful. Evidence-based guidance for older adults has argued that protein needs are commonly higher than the general adult recommendation, particularly when the goal is preservation of lean mass and function rather than merely preventing deficiency. Importantly, these recommendations are not framed as bodybuilding targets, but as pragmatic doses that better match the physiological reality of older muscle.

Another critical point is that protein's impact is not determined solely by daily totals. Distribution across meals matters because muscle protein synthesis is stimulated in a meal-responsive pattern rather than staying elevated indefinitely. Evidence from controlled human work suggests that spreading protein intake more evenly across the day can improve the overall 24-hour stimulation of muscle protein synthesis compared with patterns that concentrate most protein into one meal. This becomes especially relevant in real-world eating patterns where breakfast protein is often low and dinner protein high. If the goal is repeated stimulation of synthesis across the day, distribution becomes part of the strategy—not as diet culture advice, but as physiology.

Protein source and quality also deserve a careful, evidence-based treatment. Muscle protein synthesis depends on digestibility and essential amino acid profile, and different protein sources vary in both. Plant-based diets can support muscle health, but the evidence base often highlights practical considerations such as protein density, amino acid completeness, and achieving adequate total intake. A systematic review and meta-analysis comparing plant and animal proteins is particularly useful here, because it helps move the discussion away from ideology and into measurable outcomes in muscle mass and function.

Finally, the protein story must include training context. When resistance training is present, protein supplementation has been examined extensively for its ability to enhance training-induced gains in muscle and strength. Meta-analytic evidence indicates that additional protein—particularly when baseline intake is insufficient—can augment resistance training outcomes. This is not an argument that everyone needs supplements; rather, it clarifies that the body's response to training is partly limited by whether sufficient building blocks and signalling inputs are present.

Taken together, the evidence supports a clear framework: muscle protein synthesis is dose-responsive to protein intake, older muscle generally requires a stronger stimulus due to anabolic resistance, protein distribution can influence total daily synthesis exposure, and protein source can matter insofar as it affects amino acid availability and the ability to consistently meet requirements. From a muscle-health perspective, protein is not just another macronutrient. It is the nutritional signal most directly tied to muscle preservation across the lifespan.

Energy Availability and Macronutrient Interplay

Protein is the primary nutritional regulator of muscle protein synthesis, but it does not act in isolation. Muscle tissue operates within a wider energetic environment, and that environment determines whether protein is used for structural repair and remodelling or diverted toward meeting basic metabolic needs. Energy availability influences endocrine function, substrate utilisation, training quality, and recovery capacity. In practical terms, it sets an upper limit on how effectively muscle can adapt, regardless of how well protein intake is managed.

Energy availability and the ceiling for adaptation

Energy availability refers to the energy remaining for physiological function after the cost of exercise is accounted for. When it is adequate, the body can support recovery, tissue turnover, and adaptation. When it is chronically low, the body shifts toward conservation. This does not always prevent strength improvements, particularly early in training, but it can impair the accrual or preservation of lean mass. A meta-analysis and meta-regression examining resistance training under conditions of energy deficiency reported a consistent pattern: lean mass gains were blunted in energy deficit, even when strength outcomes were not necessarily reduced to the same degree. This distinction matters because strength can increase through neural adaptation, while lean mass change reflects the longer-term structural response. When energy is insufficient, the body may still learn to produce force more efficiently, but it becomes less willing to invest in additional contractile tissue.

This helps explain a common real-world observation: people can "get stronger" while struggling to build or maintain muscle mass when they are chronically under-fuelled. It is not that protein ceases to matter. Rather, protein operates within an energy-dependent context. When calories are too low for too long, the body increasingly oxidises amino acids for energy or reallocates them toward essential functions, narrowing the margin available for muscle remodelling.

Lean mass retention during weight loss

Energy deficit is not always accidental. Many individuals intentionally reduce calories to improve metabolic health or reduce adiposity, particularly in midlife and older age. This is where precision matters. Weight loss can improve cardiometabolic outcomes, but it can also reduce lean mass if protein intake and training stimulus are not structured appropriately. A controlled trial that combined an energy deficit with intense exercise demonstrated that higher protein intake better preserved lean mass compared with lower protein intake under the same deficit conditions. The key message is not that "more protein fixes everything," but that muscle preservation during weight loss requires both adequate protein and an adequate training signal while the body is in a catabolic environment.

This principle is also supported by more applied evidence in weight-loss settings. Work examining increased protein intake in adults with overweight or obesity pursuing weight reduction supports the practical claim that protein is a critical variable for preserving muscle tissue during dieting. When energy intake is lowered, the diet must become more deliberate, not less, because the body's default response to deficit is to downregulate costly tissue, and skeletal muscle is one of the largest and most metabolically expensive tissues to maintain.

Low energy availability as a physiological stressor

The International Olympic Committee consensus statement on Relative Energy Deficiency in Sport is important here because it frames low energy availability as a multi-system condition rather than simply a dietary mistake. When energy availability remains low for prolonged periods, physiological systems begin to adapt defensively. The IOC model describes consequences that extend beyond performance: endocrine disruption, impaired metabolic function, reduced recovery capacity, and broader health impacts. Although RED-S is most often discussed in athletic populations, it functions as a clear illustration of what chronic under-fuelling can do to the body's adaptive systems. Muscle adaptation is not isolated from those systems. When endocrine signalling and recovery capacity are compromised, maintaining or building muscle becomes harder, not because muscle "won't respond," but because the whole organism is prioritising survival over adaptation.

The relevance for general readers is straightforward. Even without meeting the formal criteria for RED-S, prolonged low energy intake, poor appetite, aggressive dieting, or high training volume without adequate intake can create a milder version of the same problem: the body begins to protect itself by reducing non-essential investment, and muscle growth and recovery become less reliable.

Carbohydrates, glycogen, and the quality of training

Carbohydrates are often treated as optional in popular nutrition debates, but their relationship with muscle function is best understood through glycogen physiology. Glycogen is the stored form of carbohydrate in skeletal muscle and liver. It supports training intensity, work capacity, and repeated high-effort contractions. The question is not whether the body can survive without carbohydrate, but whether muscle can consistently perform and adapt at a high level when glycogen availability is chronically restricted.

A review focused on carbohydrate availability and performance provides the physiological basis for why carbohydrate intake influences training outcomes. When carbohydrate availability is low, the capacity to sustain high-intensity output can be reduced, and perceived exertion often increases. This matters because muscle adaptation depends on training stimulus. If training quality drops, the mechanical signal drops with it. Even if protein intake is strong, the adaptive ceiling may still be lowered because the training stimulus is weaker.

This relationship becomes clearer when resistance training is considered directly. A systematic review and meta-analysis examining the acute effects of resistance exercise on skeletal muscle glycogen supports the idea that resistance sessions can meaningfully reduce muscle glycogen, particularly when volume is high or when multiple sets are performed near fatigue. This undermines the simplistic claim that glycogen is only relevant for endurance work. Resistance training can be glycolytically demanding, and recovery between sessions is influenced by glycogen repletion, especially for individuals training frequently or performing high-volume programs.

A glycogen-focused review further strengthens this framework by explaining glycogen's role as a performance buffer and a determinant of sustainable workload. Over time, workload is a key driver of hypertrophy and endurance adaptation. When carbohydrate intake is too low to support repeated high-quality sessions, training output can be reduced, and the cumulative stimulus necessary for adaptation may be harder to achieve.

Dietary fat and the broader energy context

Although this section focuses primarily on energy availability and carbohydrate-glycogen dynamics, dietary fat still plays an important role through total energy density and overall diet sustainability. A diet that is too low in energy can occur even when protein and carbohydrate targets appear "reasonable," especially in older adults with reduced appetite or in active individuals with high total expenditure. In that sense, dietary fat can be an important lever for maintaining adequate intake without excessive volume of food. The key point is not that fat is directly anabolic, but that maintaining adequate energy availability often requires thoughtful macronutrient balance, especially in people who struggle to eat enough.

The opposite problem: energy excess with declining muscle quality

Low energy availability is one end of the spectrum. The other end is more subtle and increasingly common: energy excess paired with low activity and poor muscle quality. This is where the concept of sarcopenic obesity becomes essential, because it challenges the assumption that higher body weight protects against muscle decline. An ESPEN and EASO consensus statement provides diagnostic framing for sarcopenic obesity and emphasises that increased fat mass can coexist with low muscle mass, low strength, and poor function. In other words, excess energy intake does not guarantee adequate muscle health. It may coexist with reduced muscle quality and higher metabolic risk.

A detailed review of sarcopenic obesity further supports the physiological plausibility of this dual condition, linking it to frailty risk, reduced physical performance, and adverse metabolic outcomes. This matters because it reinforces a core theme of this chapter: macronutrients must be understood through context. Total energy intake that exceeds needs can worsen inflammation and metabolic dysfunction, while inactivity reduces the mechanical stimulus necessary to preserve muscle. The result can be a body composition profile where total weight is high, but muscle function and resilience are low.

Putting the interplay together

Macronutrient strategy cannot be reduced to single-variable advice. Protein is essential, but it works best when energy availability is sufficient to support tissue investment.

Carbohydrates influence glycogen stores and thereby influence training quality, which influences the strength of the mechanical signal driving adaptation. Fat contributes to overall energy sufficiency and diet sustainability, particularly when appetite is low or energy demands are high. At the extremes, chronic under-fuelling impairs physiological systems that support adaptation, while chronic over-fuelling combined with inactivity can produce sarcopenic obesity, where muscle quality deteriorates despite abundant energy intake.

The practical conclusion is that optimal nutrition for muscle is not simply "high protein." It is nutritional alignment: sufficient energy to support remodelling, adequate protein to provide building blocks and anabolic signalling, and macronutrient balance that sustains performance, recovery, and metabolic health over time.

Micronutrients and the Cellular Machinery of Muscle

Macronutrients provide the bulk substrates and energy for muscle maintenance, but they do not run the machinery. The processes that allow muscle to contract, produce energy, repair tissue, and adapt to training depend on a network of vitamins, minerals, and fatty acids that act as cofactors, signalling modifiers, and structural components. When these micronutrients are insufficient, muscle function may decline even when calories and protein appear adequate. This is particularly relevant with ageing, where changes in appetite, digestion, absorption, medication use, and sun exposure increase the likelihood of subtle deficiencies.

Vitamin D and neuromuscular performance

Among micronutrients, vitamin D has one of the clearest links to muscle function and physical performance in older adults. Vitamin D receptors are present in skeletal muscle, and vitamin D status is associated with strength and mobility outcomes in ageing populations. Systematic reviews and meta-analyses examining vitamin D supplementation generally support a meaningful relationship between low vitamin D status and poorer muscle function, while supplementation tends to show the most consistent benefit in individuals who are deficient at baseline. This matters because it reframes vitamin D as a status-dependent nutrient: if levels are already sufficient, improvements may be modest, but if deficiency is present, correcting it can be functionally significant.

It is also important to distinguish standard vitamin D supplementation from active vitamin D analogues, which have been evaluated for outcomes such as muscle strength and fall risk. Meta-analytic findings in this space reinforce the broader point that vitamin D-related interventions can influence functional outcomes, but responses are variable and strongly influenced by baseline status, population characteristics, and the form of vitamin D used. The defensible conclusion is not that vitamin D is a universal strength enhancer, but that vitamin D sufficiency supports neuromuscular function, and deficiency represents a modifiable risk factor for weakness and functional decline.

Magnesium as a contractile and metabolic cofactor

Muscle contraction and relaxation rely on controlled calcium handling and ATP-dependent processes. Magnesium is central to both. It stabilises ATP, supports enzymatic reactions involved in energy metabolism, and contributes to neuromuscular stability. Reviews focusing on magnesium and muscle health in ageing populations consistently emphasise that magnesium is not simply a cramp-related mineral in popular culture; it is a core cofactor involved in the biochemistry that makes muscle work.

Evidence syntheses examining minerals in relation to sarcopenia highlight that lower magnesium intake or status is commonly associated with poorer muscle-related outcomes in older adults, although the strength of evidence varies across study designs. The safest interpretation is that magnesium adequacy supports muscle integrity and performance capacity, and that suboptimal intake becomes more consequential as the physiological buffer narrows with age. This also fits with the broader chapter theme: nutrition regulates muscle not only through protein synthesis, but through the functional efficiency of the systems that make synthesis and contraction possible.

Vitamin B12 and neuromuscular integrity

Muscle function is inseparable from the nervous system. Without adequate motor unit activation and neuromuscular signalling, muscle cannot express strength, power, or coordination effectively. Vitamin B12 is relevant here because of its role in neurological health, including pathways involved in nerve function and myelin integrity. Reviews examining vitamin B12 status in older adults link low B12 status with functional impairment, weakness, and poorer physical performance markers. Importantly, B12 deficiency risk increases with age due to reduced absorption, medication interactions, and gastrointestinal changes, meaning that deficiency can emerge even in individuals who consume animal products.

Observational and prospective evidence has also been used to explore whether B12 insufficiency predicts outcomes related to muscle mass and function, including incident sarcopenia. While these designs cannot prove causation, they strengthen a clinically relevant point: B12 status is a plausible contributor to functional decline, particularly through neuromuscular pathways. In a muscle-focused book, the value of B12 is not framed as building muscle, but as supporting the neurological foundation that allows muscle capacity to be expressed and preserved.

Omega-3 fatty acids as modulators of anabolic sensitivity and inflammation

Although omega-3 fatty acids are typically discussed as a dietary fat, their relevance to muscle health is best understood through their effects on cell membranes and signalling pathways. Systematic reviews and meta-analyses evaluating omega-3 supplementation have examined outcomes including muscle mass and strength, and in some cases indicators related to protein synthesis responsiveness. Across this literature, the most defensible interpretation is that omega-3s may support muscle health primarily by influencing inflammatory signalling and, in certain contexts, improving anabolic sensitivity—an effect that appears particularly relevant in older adults. At the same time, findings are not uniform: effect sizes vary, and some studies show minimal or no measurable benefit, highlighting that response depends on population characteristics and study design.

A consistent theme is that omega-3 supplementation tends to show the greatest promise when baseline intake is low, when inflammation or anabolic resistance may be more pronounced, or when omega-3s are combined with resistance training and adequate protein intake. In practical terms, omega-3s are best viewed as a supportive strategy that may improve the physiological environment for adaptation in selected groups, rather than a primary driver of muscle maintenance or growth.

Micronutrients as a hidden limiter of muscle outcomes

The common thread across vitamin D, magnesium, and vitamin B12 is that they influence muscle health through foundational physiology: neuromuscular signalling, contractile efficiency, and metabolic support. Omega-3s extend this framework by influencing inflammation and anabolic responsiveness. The practical implication is that muscle nutrition cannot be reduced to protein targets alone. A person can consume sufficient protein yet still experience poor outcomes if the systems that translate nutrients into function—nerve signalling, energy metabolism, and contractile processes—are constrained by micronutrient insufficiency.

This is also why deficiency and suboptimal status matter differently with age. In younger adults, a small micronutrient gap may produce minimal symptoms. In older adults, where anabolic resistance, recovery constraints, and reduced functional reserve already exist, the same gap can meaningfully alter strength, balance, fatigue resistance, and recovery capacity. In that sense, micronutrients often act as multipliers: they do not replace the primary drivers of muscle adaptation, but they influence how efficiently those drivers can operate.

Hydration, Electrolytes, and Contractile Efficiency

Hydration is often discussed as a performance variable, but for muscle tissue it is more fundamental than that. Skeletal muscle is highly water-dependent at the cellular level, and even modest fluid loss can alter physiological conditions that support contraction. Water is not simply a transport medium; it helps maintain blood volume, supports nutrient delivery, contributes to temperature regulation, and stabilises the internal environment required for repeated muscular work. When hydration status shifts, muscle performance can change with it.

Hydration status and muscle performance

Evidence examining fluid balance consistently shows that dehydration can impair exercise performance, particularly when intensity is moderate to high and repeated effort is required. In practical terms, when body water loss accumulates, perceived effort often increases and the capacity to sustain output can decline. For muscle health, this matters because adaptation depends on the quality of the training stimulus. If hydration-related fatigue reduces the ability to maintain intensity, volume, or technical control, the mechanical signal that drives adaptation may be weakened.

A critical review exploring whether fluid balance affects strength and power highlights that dehydration can negatively influence high-intensity performance outcomes, although effects vary depending on the level of dehydration, environmental conditions, and the type of task performed. More recent meta-analytic work assessing acute dehydration and indices of muscle strength supports the same general conclusion: dehydration can reduce strength-related performance, with effects becoming more likely as fluid losses increase. The defensible conclusion is not that hydration transforms strength, but that dehydration can become a limiting factor when training demands are high or conditions promote fluid loss.

Electrolytes and neuromuscular function

Hydration is not only about water volume. Muscle contraction depends on electrical excitability and the controlled movement of ions across membranes. Electrolytes—particularly sodium and potassium—help maintain membrane potentials and nerve-to-muscle signalling. During prolonged sweating, water loss occurs alongside electrolyte loss, and this combination can impair contractile efficiency and contribute to fatigue. While cramps are commonly attributed to electrolytes alone in popular discussions, the more reliable physiological framing is that fluid and electrolyte balance influences neuromuscular function and the stability of repeated contractions under stress.

Why hydration becomes more important with age

Hydration risk increases with ageing for reasons that have little to do with motivation and more to do with physiology. Older adults often experience a reduced thirst response, altered renal handling of fluid, and a higher likelihood of medication use that influences hydration status. A review focused on hydration strategies in older adults highlights that these age-related changes increase vulnerability to dehydration, particularly during heat exposure, illness, or increased activity. For muscle health, this is relevant because dehydration-related weakness, dizziness, and fatigue can reduce movement capacity, impair exercise tolerance, and indirectly increase fall risk by compromising coordination and physical stability.

Hydration as a support for recovery and training consistency

The physiological case for hydration is not limited to what happens during a workout. Training consistency across weeks and months is one of the strongest predictors of long-term muscle outcomes. Hydration supports this consistency by reducing avoidable performance decline during sessions and by supporting cardiovascular stability and thermoregulation, particularly in warm conditions. In older populations, maintaining hydration status can also influence willingness to move and exercise by reducing fatigue and discomfort associated with low fluid intake. The practical implication is that hydration is not a muscle-building tool in itself, but it can remove a preventable constraint on performance and training quality, which ultimately supports muscle preservation.

Nutrient Timing and the Adaptive Response

Nutrient timing is often marketed as a performance hack, but its real value is simpler and more physiological: it influences how often muscle receives a meaningful anabolic signal across the day. Muscle is not "building" continuously at the same rate. Instead, muscle protein synthesis rises after protein ingestion, remains elevated for a period, and then returns toward baseline. The practical question is therefore not only how much protein is consumed in total, but how frequently muscle is exposed to doses that reliably stimulate synthesis.

Timing as repeated stimulation, not a narrow window

The concept of an "anabolic window" is often presented as a short, urgent period immediately after exercise. In reality, the more defensible framing is that timing matters because it shapes the distribution of anabolic opportunities across the day. Resistance training creates a favourable environment for muscle protein synthesis, and protein ingestion provides the amino acids and signalling input needed to take advantage of that environment. But rather than relying on a single perfectly timed dose, the evidence base places more weight on regular, appropriately sized protein feedings that repeatedly stimulate synthesis.

Protein distribution across the day

One of the clearest timing questions is whether protein should be concentrated into one large meal or spread more evenly. Controlled human research has shown that distributing protein more evenly across meals can improve the overall 24-hour muscle protein synthesis response compared with patterns where most protein is consumed at a single sitting. This supports a key practical implication: if one meal contains very little protein, it may represent a missed opportunity to stimulate muscle protein synthesis that day.

A review focused on protein distribution and muscle-related outcomes reinforces this framework and highlights that distribution becomes especially relevant when total protein intake is only moderate. When total intake is already high, distribution may matter less. But when intake is borderline—common in older adults—spreading protein across meals may help increase the number of anabolic "peaks" across the day and reduce prolonged periods where muscle remains in a more catabolic balance.

Why timing becomes more relevant with age

Ageing muscle is less responsive to anabolic stimuli, meaning a stronger or more deliberate stimulus is often required to achieve the same rise in muscle protein synthesis. In this context, timing matters because it can reduce long gaps between meaningful anabolic exposures. Many older adults consume minimal protein at breakfast, moderate protein at lunch, and most of their daily protein at dinner. From a muscle physiology perspective, that pattern compresses the day's anabolic stimulation into a single event, leaving extended periods where muscle protein synthesis is not meaningfully elevated. A more even distribution—without changing total intake dramatically—can help align eating patterns with the biology of muscle turnover.

Exercise proximity and practical timing

While the narrow "window" narrative is overstated, it remains physiologically sensible to align a protein-rich meal relatively close to resistance training when possible. Training increases muscle's sensitivity to amino acids, and consuming protein in the hours surrounding a session helps ensure amino acid availability when muscle is primed for remodelling. This can be achieved without rigid rules. What matters most is that training days include sufficient total protein and that protein is not disproportionately delayed or compressed into a single late meal.

The timing principle that matters most

Across the evidence, the most defensible conclusion is that nutrient timing is valuable when it improves consistency and distribution of protein intake rather than when it creates anxiety about precise minutes. Timing should serve physiology, not perfectionism. For muscle preservation and adaptation—particularly in older adults—protein distribution across meals is one of the simplest timing strategies with plausible and supported benefits for daily muscle protein synthesis exposure.

Evidence-Based Supplementation for Muscle Health

Supplements are often presented as shortcuts, but the evidence base supports a narrower and more practical role. Supplements can be useful when they help correct a deficiency, close a gap that is difficult to meet through diet alone, or enhance training quality in specific contexts. They do not replace progressive resistance training, adequate energy intake, or sufficient daily protein, and they rarely produce meaningful changes when those foundations are absent. The most useful way to approach supplementation is therefore through an evidence hierarchy: interventions with strong support and clear relevance come first, while those with inconsistent or limited effects remain optional and context-dependent.

Creatine is the clearest example of a supplement with consistent support for muscle-related outcomes. Meta-analytic evidence in older adults indicates that creatine supplementation, particularly when paired with resistance training, can enhance gains in lean mass and strength-related measures compared with training alone. The mechanism is not mysterious. Creatine increases intramuscular phosphocreatine availability, supporting rapid ATP regeneration during high-intensity effort. That can increase training capacity—more repetitions, more total work, better maintenance of effort—and over time, greater training volume and intensity tend to produce greater adaptation. The key point is that creatine performs best as an enhancer of training output rather than as a standalone muscle-building agent.

Caffeine sits in a different category. It does not build muscle directly, but it can improve aspects of training performance by reducing perceived effort and increasing alertness and output during resistance exercise. Meta-analytic evidence supports a modest but consistent effect of acute caffeine intake on resistance exercise performance and muscular power. This matters because small improvements in training performance can compound over time if they allow higher-quality sessions. The same limitation applies here as well: caffeine is a performance tool, not a replacement for training structure or recovery. Individual tolerance, sleep sensitivity, and dose response also influence whether the benefit outweighs the trade-offs.

Beta-alanine is more specialised. Its primary role is improving buffering capacity through increased muscle carnosine, which can enhance performance during high-intensity efforts where acidosis contributes to fatigue. Systematic review and meta-analytic evidence supports its usefulness mainly in contexts requiring repeated high-intensity work over short-to-moderate durations. That means it is most relevant for certain athletic or high-volume training demands rather than general muscle preservation. In the context of muscle health across the lifespan, beta-alanine is best framed as optional and performance-specific.

BCAAs require a more cautious interpretation. They are often marketed as essential for muscle growth, but the evidence base has repeatedly questioned whether isolated BCAA supplementation adds meaningful benefit when total daily protein intake is already sufficient. Meta-analytic findings suggest BCAAs may reduce markers associated with muscle damage or soreness in certain settings, but this does not automatically translate into greater hypertrophy or strength adaptation. Where BCAAs may show more relevance is in populations with low protein intake or clinical vulnerability, but in most cases, meeting total protein requirements provides the same amino acids in a more complete and physiologically effective package. For muscle outcomes, BCAAs are therefore best viewed as situational rather than foundational.

The broader takeaway is that the strongest supplements for muscle health tend to work by improving training capacity or correcting a limiting factor. Creatine has the most consistent evidence, particularly in older adults training with resistance. Caffeine and beta-alanine may support training output in specific performance contexts. BCAAs are unlikely to outperform adequate daily protein intake for meaningful muscle adaptation. A rational supplement strategy therefore begins by identifying the bottleneck: if the bottleneck is protein intake, food or protein supplementation is the priority; if the bottleneck is training output, creatine may help; if the bottleneck is acute performance, caffeine may be useful; and if none of these bottlenecks exist, supplementation tends to have limited impact.

Conclusion

Nutrition is not a secondary consideration in muscle health. It is the biological environment in which skeletal muscle either adapts, maintains itself, or gradually declines. Throughout this chapter, we have seen that muscle outcomes are governed less by single nutrients in isolation and more by how nutritional signals interact with muscle physiology across the day, across training cycles, and across the lifespan.

Protein remains the central nutritional regulator of muscle tissue, because it supplies the amino acids required for repair and because it directly influences muscle protein synthesis. Yet even optimal protein intake operates within broader constraints. Energy availability sets a ceiling on adaptation and determines whether dietary protein is used for remodelling or diverted toward metabolic compensation. Carbohydrate and glycogen availability influence the quality and sustainability of training, shaping the mechanical signal that drives long-term adaptation. At the extremes, chronic under-fuelling compromises physiological systems required for recovery, while chronic over-fuelling paired with inactivity can coexist with declining muscle quality in the form of sarcopenic obesity.

Micronutrients then determine whether the machinery of muscle can operate efficiently. Vitamin D status influences neuromuscular function and appears most important where deficiency is present. Magnesium supports energy metabolism and contractile processes. Vitamin B12 influences neurological integrity, which underpins strength expression and coordination. Omega-3 fatty acids may support the anabolic environment in selected contexts, particularly where inflammation or anabolic resistance is more pronounced. These factors are often overlooked because they do not behave like macronutrients, but they can quietly limit function and recovery when status is low.

The chapter also clarifies that timing is not a narrow window to chase, but a question of repeated stimulation. Distributing protein across the day can increase the number of meaningful anabolic exposures, particularly in older adults who often consume protein unevenly. Hydration, while rarely framed as "muscle nutrition," can influence performance and training quality by affecting the physiological stability required for repeated contractions and sustained effort.

Finally, supplementation is best approached through evidence hierarchy rather than marketing. Creatine has the strongest support as an adjunct to resistance training, particularly in older adults. Caffeine and beta-alanine may enhance training output in specific performance contexts. BCAAs are unlikely to provide meaningful additional benefit when total dietary protein intake is adequate. Across all supplements, the consistent message is that they are amplifiers of a well-built foundation, not replacements for it.

Taken together, the scientific picture is clear. Muscle health is not preserved by a single "best" nutrient. It is preserved when nutrition aligns with physiology: sufficient protein to stimulate synthesis, adequate energy to support tissue investment, micronutrient sufficiency to maintain cellular function, and a dietary structure that supports training quality and recovery over time. When these conditions are met, skeletal muscle remains responsive, adaptable, and capable of supporting lifelong strength.

Chapter 5: Protein and Nutritional Strategy for Muscle Preservation

Introduction

Protein is often discussed as a fitness nutrient—something associated with gym culture, muscle gain, and athletic performance. But its most important role shows up later in life. As the years progress, the body becomes less efficient at maintaining lean tissue, and skeletal muscle becomes more vulnerable to gradual decline. In that context, protein is not simply a "building block." It is one of the most direct nutritional signals that determines whether muscle is preserved, repaired, and maintained at a functional level.

The reason this matters is that muscle loss is rarely dramatic in the short term. It tends to accumulate quietly across decades. A person may not notice the early shift, because everyday tasks still feel manageable. Yet the body is already moving toward a smaller physiological margin for error. Strength becomes harder to regain after illness. Recovery slows. Physical capacity narrows. By the time weakness is obvious, the decline has often been underway for years. Nutrition cannot stop ageing, but it can influence how much muscle is retained, how well it functions, and how resilient it remains.

This chapter builds on the nutritional foundations established in Chapter 4 and narrows in on protein as the central lever for muscle preservation. The goal is not to turn protein into a fad, but to explain its role with precision: how muscle uses it, how requirements shift with age, and how protein strategy can be structured in a realistic, evidence-based way. The strongest strategies are not extreme. They are consistent, repeatable, and aligned with the physiology of muscle protein turnover.

Ageing introduces a problem that is both subtle and powerful: anabolic resistance. Older muscle does not respond to dietary protein as robustly as younger muscle does. That means the same meal that once stimulated a strong rise in muscle protein synthesis may produce a smaller response later in life. Over time, this blunted responsiveness can contribute to net loss if protein intake remains low, poorly distributed, or inconsistent. The practical implication is not that older adults need to eat obsessively, but that their protein strategy often needs to be more deliberate.

This is also where the chapter remains relevant to younger adults. Muscle preservation is not something that begins at retirement age. It begins when habits are formed. Building a strong baseline of lean mass earlier in adulthood creates a larger reserve later, but maintaining that reserve still requires ongoing nutritional support. A protein strategy that supports muscle health in midlife and older age is not wasted on younger readers—it is simply an earlier investment in the same outcome: strength, resilience, and physical capability across the lifespan.

In the sections that follow, we will examine protein through a preservation lens. We will explore how muscle protein synthesis is regulated, why ageing changes protein requirements, how daily intake and distribution influence outcomes, and how protein strategy should be adapted during weight loss, reduced appetite, or periods of illness. We will also address protein sources and supplements without ideology, focusing on what the evidence supports and what is achievable in real life.

Protein as a Preservation Signal

It is tempting to think of protein as a structural material—something the body uses like bricks to rebuild muscle. That description is partly true, but it is incomplete. Protein influences muscle not only because it supplies amino acids, but because it provides the nutritional signal that governs whether muscle tissue is maintained or gradually dismantled over time. In skeletal muscle, preservation is not automatic. It is regulated.

Muscle is in constant renewal. Proteins within the contractile apparatus are continually being broken down and rebuilt, even in people who never train. This turnover allows damaged proteins to be replaced and maintains functional integrity. Whether muscle mass remains stable depends on the net balance between muscle protein synthesis and muscle protein breakdown across the day. In the fasted state, breakdown slightly exceeds synthesis. After protein ingestion, essential amino acids become available and synthesis rises, shifting the balance toward maintenance or net gain. The long-term outcome is the sum of these repeated daily cycles.

This is where protein becomes a preservation signal rather than merely a substrate. Muscle protein synthesis is not increased in a linear fashion simply because more calories are present. It is stimulated specifically by essential amino acids, and it responds most strongly when those amino acids rise to a meaningful level after a meal. Exercise amplifies this effect by sensitising muscle to amino acids, which is one reason resistance training and adequate protein intake work so effectively together. But even without exercise, protein ingestion remains one of the strongest nutritional drivers of anabolic signalling in muscle tissue.

What makes this especially important for ageing is that the default trend shifts. In younger adulthood, muscle turnover is relatively efficient. In later life, the system becomes less responsive, and the balance becomes easier to tip toward loss. A person does not need to "fail" catastrophically for this to happen. It can occur through small, repeated shortfalls: low protein at breakfast, modest intake at lunch, and reliance on one protein-heavy dinner to carry the day. Over time, this pattern reduces the number of meaningful anabolic periods and leaves muscle spending more hours in a state where breakdown is not adequately countered by synthesis.

This is also why minimum recommendations can be misleading. The minimum intake required to prevent deficiency is not necessarily the intake required to preserve muscle function and independence. Evidence-based protein recommendations for older adults consistently recognise this distinction. They emphasise that older adults often benefit from higher protein intakes than the general adult baseline, particularly when the goal is maintaining lean mass, strength, and functional capacity rather than simply avoiding malnutrition.

The most practical takeaway is that protein supports muscle in two connected ways. First, it provides essential amino acids for repair and remodelling. Second, it creates repeated anabolic signals that help keep the balance of turnover from drifting into gradual loss. This framing is important because it prevents protein strategy from becoming a trend-driven discussion about "high protein diets." Instead, it becomes a question of physiological maintenance: providing the right signal often enough to preserve muscle across time.

For younger adults, the relevance is not that protein becomes urgent, but that it becomes foundational. Building and maintaining muscle earlier in adulthood creates reserve, but that reserve is easier to maintain when protein intake supports turnover. For older adults, the relevance becomes more direct: protein strategy can meaningfully influence whether the age-related decline in muscle is mild and manageable or rapid and functionally limiting. The biology is the same across the lifespan. What changes is how much stimulus is required to produce the same result.

The Midlife Shift and Anabolic Resistance

For many people, midlife feels like a turning point in body composition. Strength becomes harder to maintain without deliberate effort, small periods of inactivity have a bigger impact, and recovery can feel slower than it did in earlier adulthood. While lifestyle factors play a major role, there is also a physiological shift occurring beneath the surface: muscle becomes less responsive to the signals that once maintained it with relatively little thought. One of the most important concepts describing this change is anabolic resistance.

Anabolic resistance refers to a reduced stimulation of muscle protein synthesis in response to protein intake and, in many cases, resistance exercise. In younger adults, a moderate protein-containing meal produces a clear rise in muscle protein synthesis, helping to counterbalance the natural breakdown that occurs between meals. With ageing, the same meal can produce a smaller anabolic response. Over time, this blunted responsiveness changes the rules of maintenance. The body does not necessarily lose muscle because protein is absent, but because the protein stimulus is no longer strong or frequent enough to generate the same protective effect.

The mechanisms underlying anabolic resistance are multifactorial, which is why the experience of muscle ageing varies between individuals. Age-related changes in muscle perfusion can reduce amino acid delivery. Chronic low-grade inflammation can interfere with anabolic signalling. There may be alterations in intracellular pathways involved in translation and muscle remodelling. Physical inactivity further compounds these changes, because disuse itself reduces anabolic sensitivity. The result is a physiological environment in which muscle requires a stronger or more deliberate signal to maintain the same tissue balance.

This is the point where protein strategy becomes critical. When anabolic resistance is present, a protein intake pattern that might have maintained muscle easily in a younger adult can become inadequate for an older adult. This is one reason why expert groups and position papers have argued for protein intakes in older adults that are commonly above the general adult baseline, particularly when the goal is preserving lean mass and function. The underlying logic is not extreme dieting; it is basic physiology: if the muscle's responsiveness is reduced, the stimulus needs to be adjusted accordingly.

Importantly, anabolic resistance does not mean older muscle is incapable of adaptation. It means the threshold for adaptation is higher and the margin for error is smaller. Older adults can still build strength and even gain muscle mass with resistance training and adequate protein, but the system is less forgiving of inconsistency. When protein intake is low, when meals are poorly distributed, or when training is sporadic, the decline accelerates. When protein and exercise are aligned consistently, muscle remains responsive and preserveable.

This is also how the chapter remains relevant to younger readers. Anabolic resistance is not an overnight event that begins at a specific birthday. It is a gradual shift that becomes more apparent over time, and it is strongly influenced by lifestyle. Building muscle earlier in adulthood increases reserve. Maintaining training habits preserves anabolic sensitivity. Establishing adequate protein intake patterns in the earlier decades reduces the likelihood of a steep drop later. The physiology that makes protein valuable in later life is the same physiology that allows muscle to adapt in youth; the difference is how much stimulus is required to produce the same return.

The practical implication is simple: midlife is the moment when protein strategy transitions from being optional to being protective. For older adults, it becomes foundational. Anabolic resistance explains why muscle decline can occur even in people who feel they are "eating normally," and it clarifies why preserving strength and independence often requires deliberate nutritional structure rather than intuition alone.

Daily Protein Targets for Maintenance and Independence

For most readers, this is the practical hinge point: how much protein is actually enough to preserve muscle as we age, and how do you choose a target that is realistic, safe, and meaningful. The answer depends on what outcome you are aiming for. The minimum intake that prevents deficiency is not the same as the intake that best supports muscle preservation, strength maintenance, recovery capacity, and long-term independence.

Expert groups that focus on ageing have repeatedly made this distinction because it reflects how muscle behaves in later life.

A useful way to approach protein targets is to separate them into three levels: a baseline for general health, a protective range for muscle preservation, and a higher range for periods of stress where muscle loss risk rises. This avoids one-size-fits-all numbers while keeping the strategy simple enough to follow.

At the general population level, many dietary guidelines still reference 0.8 g/kg/day as a broad adult baseline. However, ageing-focused position papers and clinical nutrition expert groups have argued that this level is often insufficient for preserving lean mass and function in older adults, particularly in the presence of anabolic resistance. Their recommendations shift protein targets upward because older muscle typically requires a stronger stimulus to produce a meaningful anabolic response.

For healthy older adults, a practical evidence-based target commonly recommended is around 1.0–1.2 g/kg/day. This range is not framed as extreme; it is framed as physiologically appropriate for maintaining muscle and function in later life. It also gives a buffer against the real-world reality that protein intake fluctuates day to day. Aiming for a range rather than a single number makes the approach more sustainable, especially for people who are not tracking food closely.

From a muscle-preservation perspective, the next important category is older adults who are physically active, undertaking resistance training, or trying to regain strength after a period of inactivity. In these contexts, expert guidance commonly supports protein intakes above the lower end of the older-adult range. The reason is straightforward: training increases the demand for repair and remodelling, while anabolic resistance reduces efficiency. Increasing protein intake helps close that gap, supporting better recovery and improving the likelihood that training produces a meaningful structural response.

The highest-risk category is periods of physiological stress. This includes illness, injury, hospitalisation, post-operative recovery, or any phase where appetite is reduced and physical activity drops. These periods are where older adults lose muscle fastest. Clinical nutrition guidelines in geriatrics place particular emphasis on avoiding protein inadequacy during these times, because the body shifts toward catabolism and muscle becomes a readily available amino acid source. In practical terms, many individuals do not lose independence because of ageing alone; they lose it after a medical event followed by incomplete recovery. Protein strategy becomes protective here not as a supplement trend, but as a clinical priority.

It is also important to address weight loss, because many adults in midlife and later life pursue fat loss for metabolic reasons. Energy deficit increases the risk of lean mass loss unless protein intake and training are structured deliberately. Controlled trial evidence shows that higher protein intake during an energy deficit, combined with intensive exercise, preserves lean mass more effectively than lower protein intake under similar conditions. The key takeaway is that dieting changes the rules. When calories drop, protein needs tend to rise if the goal is to preserve muscle. In older adults, this is especially important because the baseline risk of loss is already higher.

To make these targets practical, it helps to translate them into a simple method that does not require perfect tracking. The most useful approach is to pick a daily target range based on your current context and aim for consistency rather than precision.

If you are generally healthy and not currently losing weight, a reasonable protective strategy for midlife and older age is to work within the 1.0–1.2 g/kg/day range recommended by ageing-focused expert groups. If you are actively resistance training or rebuilding strength after a lull, it is often appropriate to sit toward the upper end of that range. If you are in a period of illness, recovery, or unintentional weight loss, clinical guidelines support deliberately preventing protein intake from dropping, because that is when muscle loss accelerates most quickly.

For younger adults, the same framework still applies, but the urgency is different. Younger muscle is typically more responsive, so outcomes are more forgiving when protein intake is inconsistent. Yet the long-term logic remains: the habits that make protein strategy effective in older age—adequate daily intake and reliable distribution—are the same habits that build and protect muscle reserve earlier in life. What changes with age is not the direction of the strategy, but how strongly the body depends on it.

The most defensible way to summarise daily protein targets is this: if muscle preservation and independence are the goal, protein intake should be treated as a daily input with a protective range, not a minimum to scrape past. This is especially true from midlife onward, when anabolic resistance begins to reduce the margin for error.

Distribution Across the Day

Once daily protein intake is in the right range, the next question becomes how that protein is structured. This is not a cosmetic detail. Muscle does not respond to protein intake as a slow, steady drip. Muscle protein synthesis rises after a protein-containing meal, remains elevated for a period, and then returns toward baseline. The practical implication is that protein has its strongest effect when it is consumed in doses that reliably stimulate synthesis, and when those doses occur multiple times across the day.

Many adults do not eat protein this way. A common pattern is a low-protein breakfast, a moderate lunch, and a protein-heavy dinner. From a muscle physiology perspective, this compresses most anabolic stimulation into a single late meal. It also creates long gaps earlier in the day where synthesis is not meaningfully stimulated, and the balance between synthesis and breakdown may drift toward loss. In younger adults, the system may tolerate this pattern with fewer consequences. In older adults, where anabolic resistance reduces responsiveness, the same pattern can become a meaningful limiter of preservation over time.

Controlled human research has directly examined the effect of protein distribution. Work comparing more evenly distributed protein intake across meals versus a skewed pattern has shown that distribution can positively influence 24-hour muscle protein synthesis. The significance here is not that every meal must be perfectly engineered, but that muscle appears to benefit from repeated stimulation rather than one large spike.

This concept is reinforced by broader reviews examining protein distribution and muscle-related outcomes. A key nuance is that distribution tends to matter most when total protein intake is moderate or borderline, which is often the case in older adults. If a person is already consuming high protein consistently, distribution may be less important. But when daily intake is closer to the lower end of the recommended range, spreading protein more evenly may increase the number of meaningful anabolic exposures and reduce long periods of low stimulation.

This is why distribution becomes so relevant for muscle preservation and independence. It provides a way to improve the physiological quality of a diet without necessarily increasing total intake dramatically. For example, many people can improve distribution simply by increasing protein at breakfast and slightly reducing the reliance on dinner to carry the day's intake. In older adults with lower appetite, this may also be easier than trying to consume one very large protein dose later in the day.

Distribution also matters because older adults are more likely to face practical barriers: reduced appetite, early satiety, dental issues, and a tendency to eat smaller meals. If protein is concentrated in one meal, these barriers can prevent the target from being reached reliably. Spreading protein across meals reduces dependence on any single eating opportunity and improves consistency, which is one of the strongest predictors of long-term outcomes.

A defensible way to translate this into strategy is to treat each meal as an opportunity to trigger muscle protein synthesis, rather than viewing protein as something that can be "caught up" at the end of the day. This is not about obsessing over timing. It is about increasing the number of times muscle receives an adequate anabolic signal, particularly in the decades when anabolic resistance increases the required stimulus.

The larger theme remains the same: preservation depends on repeated daily patterns. Total daily protein matters, but distribution shapes how that protein is utilised. For older adults, distribution can reduce the risk of unintentional under-stimulation. For younger adults, it provides a sustainable pattern that supports training, recovery, and the maintenance of muscle reserve over time.

Protein Quality and Source Without Ideology

Once total protein intake and distribution are addressed, the next variable is protein quality. This topic often becomes emotionally charged because it intersects with ethics, culture, and identity. But muscle physiology is indifferent to ideology. From the perspective of muscle preservation, the relevant questions are practical: how efficiently does a protein source provide essential amino acids, how well is it digested and absorbed, and how reliably can a person meet their daily target using that dietary pattern.

Proteins differ in their essential amino acid profiles and in their digestibility. Animal-derived proteins tend to provide a complete essential amino acid profile in proportions that align well with human requirements. Many plant proteins also provide valuable amino acids, but individual plant sources can vary in their amino acid composition and may be less concentrated per serving. This does not mean plant-based diets are incompatible with muscle preservation. It means that achieving equivalent physiological exposure often requires more deliberate selection, variety, and total intake.

A systematic review and meta-analysis comparing plant and animal proteins provides a useful evidence-based framing for this discussion because it focuses on measurable outcomes rather than assumptions. Across the included trials, the comparison of plant versus animal protein can be interpreted through a simple lens: when total protein intake is sufficient and diets are structured effectively, muscle-related outcomes may be more similar than popular debate suggests. When total intake is marginal or protein sources are poorly planned, differences in amino acid density and digestibility can become more influential. This is a crucial distinction for older adults, where anabolic resistance already increases the protein stimulus required for maintenance.

For muscle preservation, the key risk is not the identity of the diet but the practicality of execution. Older adults eating plant-based diets may need to pay closer attention to total protein quantity and to including a variety of higher-protein plant foods to reliably meet targets. Older adults consuming mixed diets may still fall short if their intake is inconsistent or concentrated into one meal. Protein strategy fails more often through pattern and quantity than through the label of "plant" or "animal."

Protein quality is therefore best treated as an amplifier rather than a replacement for fundamentals. Total daily intake and distribution remain the primary drivers. Protein source becomes relevant when it affects the ability to reach those targets consistently and when it influences the essential amino acid exposure needed to stimulate muscle protein synthesis in the context of ageing.

In practical terms, if someone eats a mixed diet, the goal is usually consistency rather than optimisation: reliably meeting a daily protein target and spreading it across meals tends to matter more than chasing "perfect" sources. If someone follows a plant-based diet, the same principles apply, but they may need slightly more planning to achieve adequate protein density and variety. The most important issue is not whether the diet is plant-based or animal-based; it is whether the diet delivers a reliable, repeatable protein signal strong enough to support muscle preservation over time.

Protein During Weight Loss and Metabolic Change

Weight loss is often pursued for legitimate health reasons—improved glucose control, reduced cardiometabolic risk, better joint tolerance, and improved mobility. The problem is not weight loss itself. The problem is the way weight loss commonly occurs: through calorie restriction without adequate protein intake and without a training stimulus strong enough to protect muscle. When that happens, the body does not only lose fat. It also loses lean tissue, and in midlife and older age that loss can be functionally costly.

An energy deficit shifts the body toward catabolism. Even when fat stores are available, the body also draws on amino acids to support metabolism, immune function, and glucose regulation. Muscle is the largest reservoir of amino acids in the body, and in a prolonged deficit it becomes more vulnerable to being used as a fuel source. This is why intentional dieting often leads to some degree of lean mass loss, particularly when protein intake is modest and physical activity is reduced.

For younger adults, some muscle loss during dieting may be partially regained later if training resumes and intake normalises. For older adults, the risk is greater because anabolic resistance makes regaining muscle slower and less efficient. The same dieting approach that produces acceptable outcomes at age 25 can produce a very different outcome at age 55 or 70. In these decades, muscle loss is not just a composition issue; it can translate into reduced strength, lower functional reserve, and a greater vulnerability to illness or injury.

This is where protein strategy becomes protective. Controlled trial evidence has shown that higher protein intake during an energy deficit, combined with intensive exercise, preserves lean mass more effectively than lower protein intake under similar deficit conditions. The key message is not that dieting should become protein obsession. The message is that when calories are restricted, muscle requires extra protection. Higher protein intake helps provide the amino acid availability needed to support muscle protein synthesis and reduces the degree to which muscle tissue is sacrificed during weight loss.

The same logic connects directly to Chapter 4's discussion of energy availability: adequate protein helps, but it cannot fully override the physiological pressure of a deficit. Muscle preservation during dieting therefore depends on a coordinated approach: sufficient protein intake, a resistance training stimulus, and a deficit that is not so aggressive that recovery becomes compromised. This is especially important in midlife and older age, where appetite may already be lower and training consistency may be disrupted by work, stress, or health issues.

Metabolic change adds another layer. Many adults pursue dieting in response to insulin resistance or early metabolic syndrome. Because skeletal muscle is a major site of glucose disposal, losing muscle can worsen metabolic control over time, even if short-term weight loss improves some markers. Preserving muscle during weight loss is therefore not a cosmetic goal; it is a metabolic strategy. A body that loses fat but also loses muscle may end up lighter yet less metabolically resilient.

In practical terms, the most important mindset shift is to treat weight loss as a two-part goal: reduce excess adiposity while protecting the tissue that keeps you functional. The scale can move in the "right" direction while function moves in the wrong one. A safer approach is to aim for a controlled deficit, keep protein intake deliberately high relative to body weight, and maintain some form of resistance training stimulus. For older adults, this becomes even more important because preserving independence is the outcome that matters most, and muscle is a primary determinant of that independence.

When Appetite and Intake Decline

One of the most overlooked barriers to muscle preservation in older age is not motivation or knowledge, but appetite. Many people assume muscle loss happens because older adults "stop trying," yet a more common reality is that eating enough protein becomes harder. Appetite often declines with age, meals become smaller, chewing or digestion may become more difficult, and illness can interrupt both eating and activity. When protein intake drops during these periods, muscle loss accelerates because muscle becomes an accessible source of amino acids for the body to meet basic needs.

This is why clinical nutrition guidelines in geriatrics treat protein adequacy as a priority. The concern is not only long-term "healthy eating," but the short-term risk that inadequate intake during illness, reduced mobility, or recovery periods leads to rapid functional decline. In older adults, muscle loss after a medical event can be substantial, and recovery may be incomplete if nutrition and activity are not supported. Protein strategy becomes a form of protection: it helps preserve lean tissue when the body is most likely to break it down.

Ageing-focused expert groups also emphasise that the usual adult minimums are often not enough for this stage of life. When anabolic resistance is present, the muscle-building response to protein is less efficient, which means protein intake must be more deliberate, not necessarily extreme, but structured. The challenge is that appetite decline pushes in the opposite direction. That tension—needing a stronger stimulus while wanting less food—is one of the central nutrition problems of ageing.

This is where distribution becomes more than theory. If a person struggles to eat large meals, relying on one protein-heavy meal late in the day becomes risky. It places too much pressure on a single eating opportunity, and it increases the chance that daily intake falls short. Spreading protein across smaller meals improves the likelihood of reaching the daily target and increases the number of times muscle receives a meaningful anabolic signal. Even when total intake is modest, better distribution can improve the quality of that intake from a muscle-preservation perspective.

Illness and recovery periods deserve special attention. Appetite often drops during infection, post-operative recovery, injury, or hospitalisation—exactly when muscle breakdown rises and movement decreases. Geriatric nutrition guidance treats these periods as high-risk for malnutrition and muscle loss and emphasises active prevention rather than waiting for weight loss to appear. From a preservation perspective, the goal is to avoid letting intake collapse during these episodes, because that is when the steepest losses occur.

In practical terms, if appetite is low, the priority is protein density rather than meal size. The goal is not to force huge meals, but to make the meals you do eat "count" by ensuring protein is present early and more than once per day. If breakfast is typically small, it becomes an opportunity rather than a write-off—adding a meaningful protein component there can lift total intake without requiring larger lunches or dinners.

In practical terms, if you're older and notice your intake drops during stress, sickness, or busy periods, treat that as a muscle-risk window. Don't wait until you've lost weight or feel weak. The most protective move is to keep protein intake steady during those times, even if the rest of your appetite is reduced, because muscle loss during illness is easier to prevent than it is to rebuild later.

Protein Supplements as a Tool

Protein supplements sit in a strange place in public health. They are often marketed as essential, yet for many people they are unnecessary. The evidence-based middle ground is more useful: protein supplements are tools. They are most valuable when they help someone meet a daily protein target that would otherwise be difficult to reach consistently—particularly in older adults with reduced appetite, chewing difficulty, illness-related intake decline, or time constraints that limit meal preparation. In these situations, supplements are not replacing food; they are filling a gap that carries real consequences for muscle preservation.

From a physiological standpoint, the purpose of a protein supplement is simple: to increase essential amino acid availability at a time when intake is otherwise low. If muscle preservation is the goal, the relevant outcome is not whether a protein comes from a shaker or a plate, but whether it reliably contributes to total daily protein and supports a distribution pattern that provides repeated anabolic stimulation. Because distribution becomes more important when intake is borderline—common in older populations—supplements can be particularly useful when they allow a protein-containing "meal" to exist where it otherwise would not, such as breakfast or an afternoon period where appetite is low.

The evidence base on protein supplementation is often examined in the context of resistance training. Systematic review and meta-analytic findings support the conclusion that protein supplementation can enhance gains in lean mass and strength when paired with resistance training, particularly in situations where baseline protein intake is insufficient. This matters because it clarifies what protein supplements are doing: they are not a special ingredient that bypasses physiology; they are a practical way to ensure the nutritional side of adaptation is not limiting the training response.

In clinical and geriatric nutrition guidance, the logic is even more direct. When older adults are at risk of malnutrition, frailty, or reduced intake during illness and recovery, maintaining adequate protein becomes a protective priority. In these contexts, the question becomes less about "whole foods versus supplements" and more about ensuring the body receives sufficient protein to reduce the speed and severity of muscle loss. If a supplement improves adherence to an adequate intake pattern, it is serving a clinically meaningful function.

Protein supplements also intersect with protein source preferences. People following plant-based diets can absolutely meet protein needs through food, but achieving adequate protein density can be harder when appetite is small and meal volume is limited. In those cases, plant-based protein powders can function as a practical bridge, not because plant diets are inferior, but because the real-world constraint is often volume and consistency. The same principle applies: the goal is adequate total intake and reliable distribution, regardless of dietary ideology.

It is also important to keep supplements in proportion. A protein supplement cannot compensate for chronically low total intake if it is used inconsistently, and it cannot replace resistance training as the primary mechanical signal required to maintain muscle function over time. Its role is supportive: it improves the likelihood that daily protein targets are met and that protein is distributed in a way that provides repeated anabolic stimulation—especially when appetite and intake reliability become limiting.

In practical terms, if protein intake is already consistently meeting your daily target through food, supplementation is optional. It may be convenient, but it is not necessary. If you regularly fall short—especially if breakfast is protein-light or appetite fades later in the day—using a protein supplement as a structured "bridge" can be one of the simplest ways to improve consistency without requiring larger meals.

In practical terms, if you are older or you notice your intake drops during illness, stress, or recovery periods, treat protein supplements as a temporary support rather than a lifestyle identity. The goal is not to live on shakes. The goal is to prevent avoidable drops in protein intake during high-risk periods, because muscle loss is easier to prevent than it is to rebuild later.

Conclusion

Protein strategy is often treated as optional, yet from midlife onward it becomes one of the most practical ways to protect muscle. The physiology is straightforward: skeletal muscle is continuously turning over, and whether it is maintained or lost depends on the repeated balance between muscle protein synthesis and breakdown. Protein intake influences that balance directly by supplying essential amino acids and by providing the anabolic stimulus required to preserve tissue over time. When that stimulus becomes inconsistent, muscle loss does not usually happen overnight—it accumulates quietly until functional reserve narrows.

Ageing changes the equation through anabolic resistance. As responsiveness declines, older muscle typically requires a stronger and more deliberate protein signal to achieve the same protective effect that occurred more easily in earlier adulthood. This is why expert groups focused on ageing commonly recommend protein intakes above general adult minimums when the goal is preserving lean mass and function. It is also why protein distribution matters: spreading intake across the day increases the number of meaningful anabolic exposures, which becomes especially relevant when appetite is lower and meals are smaller.

This chapter has also shown that protein strategy is not only for older adults. The habits that preserve muscle later in life are built earlier. Younger adults benefit because consistent intake supports training adaptation and maintains a higher reserve. Older adults benefit because that same consistency becomes protective, supporting strength, recovery capacity, and independence. The long-term difference is not whether someone knows protein matters, but whether their daily patterns reliably deliver enough protein, often enough, across changing life stages.

Protein strategy becomes most important when circumstances increase risk: weight loss attempts, illness, injury, and periods where intake drops and activity declines. These are the moments when muscle loss accelerates and becomes harder to regain. In these contexts, higher protein intake, deliberate distribution, and the use of protein supplements as a bridge can reduce avoidable loss and support recovery. This is not about dieting trends. It is about recognising that muscle is biologically costly tissue and therefore one of the first targets when the body is under-fuelled or under-stimulated.

In practical terms, the goal is not perfection. The goal is a repeatable protein structure that matches your stage of life. From midlife onward, protein is best treated as a daily protective input rather than a number to occasionally reach. When intake is consistent, distributed, and adequate for context, muscle preservation becomes far more achievable. When intake is erratic, low, or repeatedly deferred to one meal, the margin for error shrinks—most noticeably in the decades when independence depends on strength and reserve.

Chapter 6: Resistance Training for Lifelong Muscle Preservation

Introduction

If nutrition provides the biological environment for muscle, resistance training provides the reason for muscle to stay. Skeletal muscle is an adaptive tissue: it is maintained when it is repeatedly required, and it is downregulated when it becomes biologically "expensive" without clear demand. This is why resistance training consistently emerges as one of the most effective interventions for preserving strength, function, and independence as we age.

The relevance of this becomes clearer when we separate appearance from function. Most people do not lose independence because they "look smaller." They lose independence because strength and power fall below the threshold needed for everyday tasks—getting up from a chair, climbing stairs, catching themselves from a stumble, carrying loads, or tolerating a period of illness without steep decline. Resistance training directly targets these capacities and helps maintain the reserve that protects older adults from rapid functional loss.

Exercise guidelines reflect this reality. Major public health frameworks consistently recommend strength-building activity at least twice per week in adults, with additional emphasis on balance and functional training for older adults, because strength and stability are key determinants of fall risk and independence.

In practical terms, this chapter is not a bodybuilding manual. The goal is not maximal size or athletic performance. The goal is to explain the evidence-based principles of resistance training that preserve muscle and function across the lifespan—and to show that the "dose" required for meaningful benefit is often far more achievable than people assume.

Why Resistance Training Works

Resistance training works because it targets the primary driver of muscle retention: repeated mechanical demand. When muscle is trained against resistance, the body receives a clear signal that contractile tissue is necessary. In response, neuromuscular function improves, strength increases, and—depending on training dose and context—muscle mass and muscle quality can be preserved or improved. In older adults, this is especially important because age-related decline affects both muscle tissue and the nervous system's ability to recruit it efficiently.

The evidence for progressive resistance training in older adults is strong. A major Cochrane review found that progressive resistance training improves physical function in older people, supporting the idea that it translates beyond gym outcomes into real-world capacity. More recent evidence syntheses and reviews continue to support resistance training as an effective intervention for improving strength and functional performance and as a key component in addressing sarcopenia.

One reason resistance training is so protective is that it does not only influence muscle size. It improves the ability to produce force through improved motor unit recruitment, coordination, and rate of force development. This matters because strength declines faster than muscle mass with age, and functional capacity depends heavily on the nervous system's ability to access and express muscle capacity. Resistance training helps preserve that access.

Resistance training also supports long-term independence through its effect on task transfer. When training improves lower-body strength, trunk stability, and the ability to produce force repeatedly, everyday tasks require a smaller percentage of one's maximum capacity. That creates reserve. Reserve is what protects people when something goes wrong: a respiratory illness, a week in bed, a minor injury, or even a stressful life period that reduces activity. People with more reserve are less likely to cross the threshold into dependence.

Where the literature becomes especially useful is in clarifying that resistance training benefits are not confined to high volumes or complex programs. Network meta-analytic work examining resistance training prescriptions suggests that different combinations of variables can produce beneficial outcomes, and "optimal" training can be framed in more than one way. This supports a message that is critical for older adults: a workable program performed consistently is more valuable than a perfect program performed sporadically.

In practical terms, if you are starting later in life, the most important step is not finding the perfect routine—it is building a safe, repeatable pattern. Two sessions per week can be enough to create meaningful improvement, particularly when effort is appropriate and progression is gradual. If you are younger, the same principle applies with a different emphasis: resistance training builds reserve. The earlier that reserve is built, the more protective it becomes later.

Strength vs Power

Strength and power are often treated as interchangeable, but they are different physical qualities with different consequences for ageing. Strength is the ability to produce force. Power is the ability to produce force quickly. In day-to-day life, both matter, but power is often the missing link when we talk about independence and fall prevention.

As we age, the loss of power tends to be more functionally disruptive because so many real-world tasks require speed, not just force. Catching yourself from a trip, stepping quickly to regain balance, rising from a chair without hesitation, climbing stairs without pausing, or stabilising the trunk during an unexpected perturbation are all power-dependent tasks. If force production is slow, the body may still be "strong enough" in a maximum sense, but not fast enough to respond when timing matters.

This distinction is reflected in the research comparing power-focused training to traditional strength training in older adults. Systematic reviews and meta-analyses examining adults around 60 years and above have found that power training can produce meaningful improvements in functional outcomes, and in some contexts may outperform traditional strength-only approaches for certain measures of physical function. The key message is not that strength training stops working. It does. The message is that training strategies that include an intent to move with speed—while still controlling technique and safety—can better target the rapid force capacity that declines with ageing.

The relevance to falls risk is especially important. Falls are not simply a balance problem; they are a recovery problem. The body must detect instability and respond quickly enough to prevent a loss of base of support. Evidence syntheses linking power-oriented training to fall-risk-related functional capacity strengthen the argument that preserving rapid force production is not an athletic luxury—it is a practical protective factor in older age.

None of this suggests older adults should train recklessly or chase speed for its own sake. Power training in the evidence base is typically performed with controlled technique, appropriate loads, and emphasis on intent and acceleration rather than maximal velocity at any cost. When appropriately programmed, it can be integrated safely alongside traditional strength training. In many cases, the most realistic approach is not "either/or," but both: build force capacity and preserve the ability to express that force quickly.

In practical terms, if you are older and training only slowly with light resistance, you may still benefit, but you may not be adequately challenging the capacity that protects you during fast, unpredictable events like slips or trips. Adding carefully controlled power emphasis—such as rising from a chair with purposeful speed, or performing the lifting phase of a resistance exercise with more intent while keeping the lowering phase controlled—can help train the quality that is most vulnerable to ageing. For younger adults, the message is preventative: training that includes both strength and power builds a broader reserve, and that reserve is what protects function when age-related decline eventually begins.

The Minimum Effective Dose Approach

One of the biggest barriers to resistance training in midlife and older age is not willingness, but perceived complexity. Many people assume that meaningful results require long sessions, complex programming, or an athlete's schedule. The evidence does not support that assumption. A more useful framework—especially for muscle preservation—is the minimum effective dose: the smallest amount of resistance training that still produces meaningful improvement in strength and function. For older adults, this framing matters because the goal is not optimisation for sport. The goal is maintaining capacity reliably enough to protect independence.

Reviews examining minimal dose training consistently show that strength can increase with relatively low volumes of resistance exercise, particularly in individuals who are untrained or returning after time off. Early gains are often driven by improved neuromuscular coordination and more efficient force production rather than large increases in muscle size. This is encouraging because functional outcomes are often linked to strength and power capacity, not simply visible hypertrophy. It also means that a realistic program, performed consistently, can produce protection even when time and energy are limited.

Minimal dose does not mean minimal effort. It means minimal volume with meaningful stimulus. In practice, this usually involves training major movement patterns consistently with enough load or intensity that the muscles are challenged and adaptation is required. Evidence-based discussions of minimal dose training emphasise that frequency and effort interact. A smaller amount of training performed with appropriate effort can still produce gains, particularly when progression occurs over time.

For muscle preservation, the most important concept is consistency across months and years. Many people fall into a cycle of overreaching, soreness, long breaks, and restarting. This pattern is common in older adults who attempt to "make up for lost time" with a burst of intensity. Minimal dose strategies help reduce that boom–bust cycle by making training sustainable. A small, repeatable amount of resistance training—performed week after week—generally produces more protection than occasional high-volume phases separated by inactivity.

This framework also supports younger readers. Minimum effective dose is not a ceiling; it is a floor. For someone who wants to build more muscle and strength, training volume may be higher. But understanding the minimum dose is valuable because it removes the all-or-nothing mindset. Even during busy periods, a minimal program can maintain strength and muscle, preserving the reserve that supports long-term outcomes.

In practical terms, if you are starting in midlife or older age, the simplest minimum effective dose is often two resistance training sessions per week targeting the major movement patterns, performed with controlled technique and gradually increasing challenge over time. If life becomes busy or health interrupts training, aim to maintain at least one session per week rather than stopping completely, because the consistency of exposure is what preserves adaptation. For older adults, this approach is often safer, more sustainable, and more protective than attempting to train like a younger athlete without the recovery capacity to match.

Progression Without Injury

For resistance training to preserve muscle over the long term, it must be progressive. If the stimulus never increases, the body adapts and then stabilises. But progression does not mean constant escalation or pushing to failure in every session.

Especially in midlife and older age, the most sustainable form of progression is gradual, planned, and compatible with recovery capacity. The goal is not to "train hard" in a short burst. The goal is to keep training possible and productive for decades.

The evidence base on resistance training variables consistently supports the idea that multiple loading strategies can improve strength and hypertrophy. What matters is not a single perfect load or repetition range, but that training provides sufficient mechanical tension and effort to drive adaptation, and that this stimulus is increased over time. Reviews on loading recommendations emphasise that heavier loads are particularly effective for maximising strength, while a broader range of loads can contribute to hypertrophy when sets are performed with sufficient effort. For muscle preservation, the practical implication is reassuring: progression can occur through different routes. It does not require extreme weights, but it does require that training remains challenging.

In midlife and older age, the limiting factor is often not muscle, but connective tissue tolerance. Tendons, joint structures, and recovery processes may respond more slowly to sudden increases in training load or volume. This is why many people get injured not because resistance training is unsafe, but because progression was too aggressive or too inconsistent. Reviews focused on optimising strength training strategies emphasise the importance of appropriate progression and recovery rather than simply increasing load as fast as possible.

Progression also includes more than weight. It can occur through increasing repetitions with the same load, adding an additional set, improving technique and range of motion, increasing training frequency, or reducing rest periods in a controlled way. For older adults, these forms of progression can often be more joint-friendly than rapid increases in absolute load. The body still receives a stronger stimulus, but the increase is more tolerable.

The most common progression mistake in older beginners is treating discomfort as a sign that training is wrong, rather than as a signal that progression needs to be adjusted. Soreness after unfamiliar exercise is normal, but persistent joint pain, sharp discomfort, or pain that worsens session to session should be treated as feedback. When training is progressed at an appropriate rate, the body adapts not only in muscle but also in connective tissues, improving capacity over time.

In practical terms, a safe progression mindset is to aim for steady improvement without urgency. If you can add a small amount of load, a repetition, or a set over time while keeping technique stable and recovery manageable, you are progressing. For midlife and older adults, the goal is to finish sessions feeling challenged but not destroyed, because the ability to train again consistently next week matters more than a single heroic workout. If something feels irritated, reduce the progression step rather than abandoning training altogether. This is how resistance training stays protective rather than becoming a cycle of flare-ups and restarts.

Exercise Selection That Transfers to Life

The question "What exercises should I do?" often gets answered with gym culture rather than physiology. For muscle preservation and independence, exercise selection is best guided by transfer: does the training improve the movements and capacities that determine daily function and reduce risk when something goes wrong? In older age, that usually means protecting the ability to stand up, climb, carry, stabilise, and recover balance. In midlife, it means maintaining those capacities so that decline is slower and interruptions (injury, illness, busy years) do not create disproportionate loss.

Resistance training guidelines and position statements consistently emphasise training the major muscle groups, using multi-joint movements where appropriate, and integrating balance-related work in older adults. The reason is not that isolation exercises are "bad," but that whole-body patterns are efficient, and they map more closely to real-world tasks. When the training signal is limited by time, fatigue tolerance, or joint considerations, it makes sense to prioritise the movements that deliver the most functional return.

A useful way to organise exercise selection is by movement patterns rather than by body-part splits. This keeps the focus on function, not aesthetics. The core patterns that tend to transfer best to daily life include squatting, hinging, pushing, pulling, carrying, and locomotion, with balance and stepping work layered in for older adults. These are not special "functional exercises." They are the basic ways humans interact with the physical world: rising and lowering, picking things up, reaching and pushing objects away, pulling objects toward the body, holding loads while moving, and reacting to instability. Training these patterns strengthens the muscular and neuromuscular systems in a way that naturally supports everyday competence.

Lower-body patterns are especially important because lower-body strength and power are strongly tied to mobility and fall resilience. Rising from a chair is essentially a squat pattern. Stair climbing combines repeated knee and hip extension with balance control. Getting up from the floor involves coordinated lower-body and trunk effort. When older adults lose these capacities, independence narrows quickly because daily movement becomes costly and fatigue rises. Resistance training that prioritises lower-body patterns therefore offers a direct functional return, particularly when training also includes power emphasis as discussed earlier in the chapter.

Upper-body patterns matter for independence in a different way. Carrying shopping bags, lifting objects into cupboards, pushing up from a chair or bed, opening heavy doors, pulling objects closer, and stabilising while reaching all rely on upper-body strength and trunk control. Upper-body weakness can also indirectly increase fall risk: when balance is lost, the ability to grab a rail, catch oneself, or stabilise the trunk can reduce the severity of a stumble. This is one reason guidelines for older adults do not focus only on legs; they emphasise whole-body strength and balance.

Exercise selection also needs to respect a reality that becomes more common with age: joint limitations. Many midlife and older adults have knee discomfort, hip stiffness, shoulder issues, or spinal sensitivity. The goal is not to "push through" in a way that escalates pain and leads to dropout. The evidence base supporting resistance training in older adults includes a wide range of modalities and intensities, which implies something important: there is rarely only one correct exercise. There are multiple ways to train the same pattern. A squat pattern can be trained with a chair sit-to-stand, a goblet squat, a leg press, or a supported squat variation. A hinge can be trained with a hip hinge drill, a Romanian deadlift with light load, a kettlebell deadlift from an elevated start, or a hip extension variation. This flexibility makes resistance training far more accessible and sustainable across ageing populations.

Another important element of exercise selection is simplicity. Complex exercises are not automatically better. Many older adults benefit more from movements they can repeat consistently with good technique than from constantly changing variations. Consistency improves skill, confidence, and progression. Skill matters because neuromuscular improvements are a major part of strength gains, especially early in training, and maintaining skill is part of preserving reserve. When movement patterns are practised reliably, the nervous system maintains coordination and recruitment efficiency, which supports strength expression and reduces the "rust" that builds when training is sporadic.

Balance and stepping deserve a deliberate place in this chapter, because transfer to life is not only about strength. Falls prevention evidence supports exercise as a key intervention, and guidelines commonly recommend balance-focused activity for older adults alongside strength training. Balance is not purely inner-ear function; it is also strength, reaction time, coordination, and confidence. Strength training contributes to balance resilience by increasing the capacity to control the body, but adding balance-specific exposure—controlled stepping, single-leg stance work, changing direction, and similar tasks—helps train the specific skill of stability under dynamic conditions.

In practical terms, if someone is building a simple resistance training routine for muscle preservation, the easiest way to choose exercises is to cover the main patterns and repeat them long enough to progress. For many adults, that means selecting a squat pattern, a hinge pattern, a push, a pull, and a carry variation across the week, and then adjusting the exact exercise choice to suit joints and equipment. If you are older, include at least one balance or stepping component regularly, even if it is brief, because strength and balance together are more protective than either alone. The goal is not variety for its own sake—it is functional return with a plan you can sustain.

Recovery and Adaptation in Midlife and Older Age

A resistance training program is only as effective as the recovery that follows it. Adaptation does not occur during the workout itself; it occurs in the hours and days afterward as the body repairs tissue, restores energy systems, and remodels neuromuscular function in response to the stimulus. With ageing, the need to respect recovery becomes more important—not because older adults are fragile, but because the cost of recovery tends to rise and the penalty for poorly managed training is often a longer interruption. In a muscle preservation context, interruptions matter because consistency is one of the strongest predictors of long-term outcomes.

Ageing changes recovery in several ways that influence how training should be structured. Muscle protein synthesis response becomes less efficient with age unless nutrition is supportive, and connective tissue tolerance may adapt more slowly. Sleep quality often declines in midlife and later life, which can affect perceived recovery and readiness to train. Older adults may also carry more joint pathology or movement restrictions, which means that training stress accumulates faster and tissue irritation can become limiting if progression is too aggressive. None of these factors rule out hard training; they simply mean that training needs to be intelligently dosed. Position statements on resistance training in older adults emphasise that older individuals respond well to training, but also that programming should consider recovery capacity, progression rate, and long-term adherence.

The most common mistake in midlife and older age is oscillating between too much and too little. People often train intensely after a gap, become excessively sore or flare a joint, then stop for weeks, then restart from scratch. This creates a repeating cycle of deconditioning and reconditioning rather than stable adaptation. Minimal effective dose strategies exist partly to prevent this pattern. A smaller, consistent training dose that is repeated across months will generally outperform sporadic "hero sessions," particularly when the goal is preservation rather than maximal performance. Reviews on minimal dose training reinforce that meaningful gains can occur without high volumes, which supports a recovery-friendly approach that keeps training sustainable.

Recovery is also influenced by how training variables are manipulated. Load, volume, and effort can all drive adaptation, but they also drive fatigue. Reviews on loading and training strategy highlight that there are multiple effective ways to train. For older adults, this flexibility is useful because it allows training to be progressed without pushing every variable simultaneously. For example, a person may maintain load but reduce volume during a stressful week, or focus on technique and range of motion improvements rather than chasing heavier weights during periods of low sleep. This approach keeps the training signal present while controlling the recovery cost.

Another important recovery principle is spacing. Most guidelines and expert recommendations support resistance training at least twice per week for older adults, but this does not mean training the same pattern hard on consecutive days. Many people do better with sessions spaced across the week, allowing recovery of the trained tissues while still maintaining enough frequency for adaptation and skill retention. This is especially true when power-focused work is included. Power training requires freshness and coordination, so recovery and readiness matter as much as load selection. Meta-analyses comparing power and strength training reinforce that both can improve function, but they also imply that power outcomes depend heavily on quality of execution. That quality is harder to achieve when fatigue is high.

The role of recovery also explains why some individuals feel "worse" when they begin training after years of inactivity. The first few weeks often carry delayed onset muscle soreness and a sense of fatigue as tissues adapt to new demands. This is not a sign that training is harmful; it is a sign that the body is unaccustomed to the stimulus. The key is to begin at a dose the body can recover from and progress gradually. When the initial dose is too high, the soreness and fatigue can create a negative feedback loop where training is associated with discomfort and drop-out becomes more likely.

Finally, recovery is not separate from nutrition. Chapter 4 and 5 established that adequate energy and protein support adaptation and reduce the risk of excessive lean mass loss, especially under stress. For older adults, protein distribution and overall intake help support the anabolic environment needed to recover from training. Resistance training and nutrition are therefore not parallel strategies; they are cooperative. Training creates the stimulus, and nutrition supports the rebuilding.

In practical terms, the simplest recovery strategy for midlife and older adults is to prioritise consistency over intensity spikes. Aim for sessions that are challenging but leave you able to train again reliably next week. If soreness persists or joints become irritated, adjust one variable at a time—reduce volume, reduce load, or modify the exercise—rather than abandoning training altogether. If life becomes chaotic, keep a minimal dose routine rather than stopping completely, because maintaining exposure protects neuromuscular skill and slows detraining. For muscle preservation, the most protective training plan is the one you can keep doing.

When Training Isn't Possible

No matter how well a training plan is designed, life will interrupt it. Illness, injury, surgery, flare-ups of joint pain, travel, caregiving demands, or simply overwhelming schedules can temporarily remove access to structured resistance training. For muscle preservation, the goal during these periods is not to pretend that detraining doesn't happen. The goal is to reduce the *rate* of loss, protect function, and make returning to training smoother and safer.

A useful way to think about interruptions is that muscle and strength are not lost at the same rate, and they are not rebuilt at the same rate either. Early losses in strength during a break are often driven by changes in neuromuscular efficiency, coordination, and reduced exposure to the movement patterns you've been practising. This is one reason people can feel "weaker" surprisingly quickly even if muscle size has not changed much. Over longer interruptions, loss of lean tissue can become more relevant, especially when activity levels drop and appetite or protein intake declines at the same time. The more complete the interruption, the faster the drift.

This is where the "minimum effective dose" principle becomes protective in a different way. Earlier in this chapter, minimum effective dose was presented as a way to make training sustainable. During interruptions, it becomes a way to preserve adaptation with a smaller input than people assume is necessary. Reviews on minimal dose resistance training show that strength can be maintained or improved with relatively low volumes, particularly when the exercises are performed with adequate effort and consistency. That does not mean one workout will preserve everything indefinitely, but it does mean that maintaining *some* form of resistance exposure can dramatically change the trajectory compared with stopping completely. The body responds strongly to continued signals of demand, even if that signal is smaller than your usual routine.

In older adults, this matters because interruptions often coincide with the very events that accelerate muscle loss: bed rest, reduced mobility, reduced appetite, and recovery periods. In these contexts, muscle preservation becomes less about "fitness" and more about preventing a step down in baseline capacity that never fully returns. Position statements and guidelines for older adults consistently emphasise resistance training because it supports functional capacity, and that same logic applies during recovery phases: keeping some degree of muscular demand present helps preserve the capacity that protects independence.

When training truly isn't possible—for example, after surgery or during acute illness—the next best target is maintaining movement and function within medical limits. Even low-level activity can help preserve coordination, circulation, and confidence in movement. The key is not intensity; it is avoiding prolonged total inactivity when safe alternatives exist. This is especially relevant for older adults because the longer the period of complete inactivity, the harder it can feel to restart, and the greater the risk that fear of movement becomes an additional barrier.

The return-to-training phase also deserves careful attention. The most common mistake after a break is restarting at the previous workload. Tissues decondition during interruptions, and recovery capacity can be lower than expected. A safer approach is to treat the first few sessions back as re-entry: focus on technique, controlled ranges of motion, and conservative loading, then rebuild progressively. This is where the long-term strategy matters. People who have a simple, repeatable routine and understand progression tend to return more smoothly than those who rely on sporadic bursts of effort.

The final piece is that interruptions in training often come with changes in eating. During illness or stress, protein intake frequently drops. Appetite decreases, meal patterns become irregular, and convenience choices replace structure. In earlier chapters we established that muscle preservation is the combination of mechanical stimulus and nutritional support. When training is reduced, maintaining protein becomes even more important because the body is more likely to drift into a negative protein balance. The aim is not perfection, it is simply preventing avoidable drops in protein intake during high-risk periods.

In practical terms, if you can't do your full routine, aim to keep a "bridge routine" rather than stopping completely. One short session per week, or even a brief set of key movement patterns performed at home, can help preserve skill and strength far better than an all-or-nothing stop. If you are older, the priority is often lower-body patterns and safe balance-related movement because these are most closely tied to independence.

In practical terms, if you return after a break, restart below your previous level even if you feel impatient. Build back over weeks, not days. If you treat re-entry as part of the plan rather than a failure, interruptions become manageable rather than disastrous. And during any period of reduced activity, keep protein intake as steady as you reasonably can—because preventing muscle loss is always easier than rebuilding it later.

How Nutrition Supports Training Outcomes

Resistance training provides the mechanical signal that preserves muscle, but nutrition determines how effectively the body can respond to that signal. Training creates stress, microdamage, and a demand for remodelling. Nutrition supplies the substrates needed to repair tissue and the signals that regulate whether muscle protein synthesis rises enough—and often enough—to produce long-term preservation.

Protein remains the central nutritional variable. Resistance exercise sensitises muscle to amino acids, and adequate protein intake supports the rise in muscle protein synthesis that follows training. This is particularly important from midlife onward, when anabolic resistance reduces responsiveness and the margin for error narrows. When protein intake is consistently low or poorly distributed, training still helps, but the structural response can be limited. When protein intake is adequate and distributed across the day, training outcomes become more reliable and recovery tends to improve. In practical terms, training provides the reason for muscle to stay, but protein provides the resources and signal to maintain it.

Energy availability is the next layer. If energy intake is chronically insufficient, the body is more likely to use amino acids as fuel and less likely to invest in tissue remodelling. Under-fuelling can also reduce training quality by increasing fatigue and reducing work capacity, which weakens the mechanical stimulus driving adaptation. For older adults, this matters because appetite is often lower and energy deficits may occur unintentionally, especially during illness or stressful life periods. Adequate energy intake does not guarantee muscle preservation, but chronic inadequacy can quietly undermine it.

Micronutrients and hydration support the machinery that makes training possible. Vitamin and mineral sufficiency influences neuromuscular function, energy metabolism, and tissue repair processes. Hydration supports cardiovascular stability, temperature regulation, and contractile efficiency, which affects training quality and tolerance. These factors rarely replace the primary drivers of adaptation, but they can become hidden constraints when status is low—especially in older adults where recovery capacity is already more limited.

Finally, nutrition supports consistency. Resistance training only protects muscle if it is repeated over time. Nutrition contributes to this by supporting recovery, reducing excessive fatigue, and helping people feel capable of training again. When training and nutrition are aligned, the system becomes self-reinforcing: strength improves, daily tasks become easier, activity increases, and maintenance becomes more sustainable.

In practical terms, the simplest integration is to treat training and nutrition as a paired system. If you are committing to resistance training, make protein intake a daily constant rather than something that varies wildly. Aim to avoid aggressive under-eating that leaves you drained and inconsistent. If you are older, treat periods of illness or low appetite as moments to protect intake rather than let it collapse, because those are the periods where muscle loss accelerates most quickly. When the mechanical signal and the nutritional signal are both present, muscle preservation becomes far more achievable.

Conclusion

Resistance training is not simply an optional fitness activity. It is one of the most reliable interventions we have for preserving muscle function, strength, and independence as we age. Muscle is biologically expensive tissue. When it is regularly required, the body maintains it. When it is consistently underused, the body downregulates it. Resistance training provides a clear mechanical reason for muscle to stay, and it does so in a way that directly improves the capacities that determine daily function.

This chapter has shown that muscle preservation is not only about size. Strength and power are the functional currencies that protect independence. Strength supports tasks like rising from a chair, climbing stairs, and carrying loads. Power—force produced quickly—often becomes even more critical for real-world safety because it underpins balance recovery and fall resilience. Evidence comparing power-focused training with traditional strength training reinforces that including an intent to move with speed, when performed safely and appropriately, can improve functional outcomes that matter in later life.

Perhaps the most encouraging message is that meaningful benefit does not require extreme programs. The minimum effective dose concept helps remove the all-or-nothing mindset that keeps many adults from starting or staying consistent. Strength and functional gains can occur with relatively low volumes when training is performed with adequate effort and progressed gradually. This is especially valuable in midlife and older age, where sustainability matters more than perfection and where avoiding injury and long interruptions is part of the preservation strategy.

Progression remains necessary, but it must be intelligent. The goal is not constant escalation; it is steady development that respects connective tissue tolerance and recovery capacity. Exercise selection also matters most when it transfers to life. Training major movement patterns and including balance-relevant exposure in older age supports the physical competencies that reduce dependence and improve resilience. When interruptions occur—and they will—the most protective approach is not to abandon training, but to reduce to a workable minimum and return gradually.

Finally, resistance training works best when it is supported by nutrition. Adequate protein and sufficient energy availability help translate training stimulus into repair and remodelling, particularly as anabolic resistance increases with age. Training and nutrition are not competing strategies. They are cooperative inputs in the same preservation system.

In practical terms, the long-term message is simple: treat resistance training as a foundational habit of healthy ageing. The objective is not to train like an athlete. The objective is to protect the capacity that keeps life accessible—movement, stability, recovery, and independence. When resistance training is applied consistently and supported appropriately, muscle remains remarkably adaptable across the lifespan, and ageing becomes far more likely to be accompanied by capability rather than progressive limitation.

Chapter 7: Nutrition Patterns for Muscle Preservation

Introduction

Nutrition for muscle preservation is often discussed through individual nutrients: protein, amino acids, supplements, vitamins, minerals, and hydration. Those details matter, and earlier chapters have explained why. But in real life, people do not eat nutrients in isolation. They eat meals, snacks, habits, routines, and patterns repeated over months and years. Those patterns determine whether the body consistently receives the support it needs to maintain muscle, recover from training, regulate metabolism, and remain resilient with age.

This chapter moves from isolated nutrition principles into the broader structure of eating. The goal is not to prescribe one perfect diet or force every reader into the same food choices. A muscle-preserving dietary pattern can look different from person to person depending on culture, preference, budget, appetite, health status, and daily routine. What matters is whether the pattern reliably supports the same core outcomes: adequate protein, sufficient energy, useful micronutrients, fibre-rich whole foods, and a lower reliance on foods that displace nourishment without supporting long-term function.

This is especially important from midlife onward. As anabolic resistance increases, appetite may change, recovery can become less forgiving, and periods of inactivity or illness can have a greater effect on muscle. Under those conditions, a diet that is technically adequate on some days but inconsistent overall may not provide enough repeated support. Muscle preservation depends less on occasional ideal meals and more on whether the usual pattern is strong enough to hold up under ordinary life.

Diet quality also matters because muscle does not exist separately from metabolic health, inflammation, gut function, and recovery. A higher-quality pattern can make it easier to manage these systems at once, while a diet dominated by ultra-processed foods may provide plenty of calories but still leave the body poorly supported. This distinction is important: the issue is not food purity, but nutritional direction. A diet can be flexible and enjoyable while still being structured enough to protect muscle.

In the sections that follow, we will examine what a muscle-preserving dietary pattern looks like in real life. We will look at Mediterranean-style and high-quality eating patterns, the effect of ultra-processed foods on diet quality, the importance of protein distribution across meals, the role of fibre and whole foods, and how these principles shift across midlife and older age. The aim is to give the reader a practical framework that can be repeated, adjusted, and sustained over time.

Designing a Muscle-Preserving Diet Pattern in Real Life

A muscle-preserving way of eating does not need to be rigid, fashionable, or built around perfect food choices. In practice, the most protective dietary patterns tend to share a few key traits. They make it easier to eat enough total protein, distribute that protein more effectively across the day, maintain adequate overall energy intake, and obtain fibre and micronutrients from largely whole or minimally processed foods. They also reduce reliance on foods that are easy to overconsume yet poor at building a strong nutritional foundation.

This matters because muscle preservation is shaped by the total dietary environment, not simply by the presence or absence of one nutrient. A person can technically eat enough protein on paper while still following a pattern that is inconsistent, under-fuelled, fibre-poor, or heavily dependent on ultra-processed foods. Over time, that kind of pattern can work against the broader conditions that support muscle maintenance, recovery, metabolic health, and physical function. A stronger pattern does more than include protein. It creates a nutritional setting in which adequate protein intake is more likely to be achieved and used effectively.

One useful way to think about this in daily life is to build meals around anchors rather than rules. A meal that supports muscle usually contains a meaningful protein source, some form of plant food, and enough total food to be genuinely nourishing rather than tokenistic. That can look very different depending on culture, food preferences, budget, and appetite, but the principle remains stable. Muscle-preserving diets are not defined by one cuisine or one ideal menu. They are defined by whether they reliably support nutritional adequacy and consistency over time.

Mediterranean-style eating is often used as a useful model, not because everyone must eat in a Mediterranean way, but because this pattern tends to combine several favourable characteristics at once. It generally includes legumes, vegetables, fruit, whole grains, olive oil, nuts, fish, yoghurt or other dairy foods, and fewer heavily processed convenience products. From a muscle perspective, that combination is useful because it supports overall diet quality while also making it easier to achieve better protein intake, better carbohydrate quality, and a broader intake of nutrients associated with healthy ageing. Its value lies less in the label and more in the structure.

A practical muscle-preserving pattern also avoids the common habit of making dinner the only nutritionally serious meal of the day. In many real-world diets, protein intake is heavily concentrated in the evening, while breakfast and lunch contribute relatively little. That pattern is understandable, but it is not ideal. When most protein is pushed into one meal, the day becomes nutritionally uneven. A more effective approach is one in which each main meal contributes meaningfully, even if intake is not perfectly identical from meal to meal.

This does not mean every meal must be precisely balanced. It means the overall day should not repeatedly drift into long stretches of low intake followed by a late attempt to make up for it. For older adults especially, that strategy becomes less reliable because appetite may be lower, portion tolerance may be reduced, and anabolic responsiveness may be less robust than it was earlier in life. A dietary pattern that depends too heavily on one large evening meal is often less realistic than one that spreads nutritional value more evenly across the day.

Fibre also has an important place in this conversation, not because it is the main focus of muscle nutrition, but because fibre-rich foods are often markers of better overall dietary quality. Diets rich in legumes, vegetables, fruit, and whole grains usually bring more than fibre alone. They also tend to provide a wider micronutrient profile and displace a greater proportion of low-value, ultra-processed foods. That matters because a person may meet protein targets while still eating in a way that is unnecessarily narrow and metabolically less supportive over the long term.

At the same time, a muscle-preserving diet should not become so idealised that it stops being practical. Diet quality matters, but so does adherence. If an eating pattern is too restrictive, too expensive, too time-consuming, or too dependent on constant food preparation, it becomes harder to sustain. A useful pattern is one that survives ordinary life: work, family pressure, fluctuating appetite, social eating, periods of illness, and days when motivation is low. Durability matters. The best dietary pattern for muscle is not the one that looks most impressive on paper. It is the one that can be repeated consistently for years.

In practical terms, the goal is not dietary perfection. It is repeatable structure. Most main meals should contain a clear source of protein. Most days should include a reasonable intake of plant foods. Most of the diet should come from foods that still resemble their original ingredients. Convenience foods can still have a place, but they should support the pattern rather than dominate it.

In practical terms, adults trying to preserve muscle should pay close attention to what their usual eating pattern makes easy and what it makes difficult. If breakfast is almost always low in protein, that matters. If lunch is regularly skipped, that matters. If most food comes from packets, takeaway meals, or heavily processed snack foods, that matters too. The issue is not moral judgment. The issue is whether the pattern reliably supports muscle tissue, recovery, and function.

In practical terms, flexibility should be seen as a strength rather than a compromise. Different people may rely on yoghurt, eggs, dairy, legumes, tofu, fish, meat, or protein-fortified foods to help build the same overall pattern. The details can vary. What should remain stable is the overall direction: regular protein, adequate intake, better-quality staples, and less dependence on foods that crowd out nourishment.

The Role of Mediterranean-Style and High-Quality Dietary Patterns

When researchers study nutrition and muscle health at the whole-diet level, one pattern appears again and again: the higher-quality pattern built around minimally processed foods, adequate protein, plant variety, and overall nutritional balance. Among named dietary models, the Mediterranean-style pattern is the one most consistently associated with better ageing outcomes, including lower frailty risk and, in many studies, more favourable muscle-related outcomes. This does not mean it is a magic formula, nor does it mean every traditional Mediterranean diet is identical. What matters is that it tends to bring together several features that support muscle preservation at the same time.

That combination is important. Muscle is affected not only by protein intake, but by the broader nutritional environment in which protein is consumed. A high-quality dietary pattern usually improves the likelihood of adequate total energy intake, better protein sources, better micronutrient exposure, and a lower reliance on foods that displace nourishment. In that sense, the Mediterranean-style pattern is useful less because it is culturally branded and more because it is structurally sound.

What High-Quality Eating Usually Includes

High-quality dietary patterns are usually built around foods that still look like food. They tend to include vegetables, fruit, legumes, whole grains, nuts, seeds, olive oil or other unsaturated fat sources, dairy foods or equivalent alternatives where appropriate, and regular inclusion of protein-containing foods such as fish, eggs, yoghurt, milk, legumes, poultry, meat, or soy-based foods. These patterns do not need to exclude enjoyment, but they are generally less dependent on ultra-processed products as the default foundation of the diet.

From a muscle-preservation perspective, this matters because these foods do more than provide isolated nutrients. They help shape the daily pattern in a way that makes adequate intake more achievable. A meal pattern built from yoghurt, oats, fruit, legumes, eggs, fish, grains, vegetables, and dairy, for example, is more likely to support protein adequacy and overall nutritional sufficiency than one built mainly from snack foods, refined convenience products, and energy-dense packaged meals.

This is also one reason high-quality patterns tend to outperform nutrient-focused thinking. Real diets are not built from protein alone. They are built from combinations of foods that either work together well or work against each other. When the overall pattern is stronger, many individual nutritional problems become easier to solve.

Why It Matters for Ageing Muscle

Ageing muscle responds best to consistency. It benefits from a dietary pattern that repeatedly supplies enough nourishment to support maintenance, repair, and adaptation. High-quality dietary patterns appear to help here because they reduce the likelihood of several common nutritional problems occurring at once. They make it less likely that protein intake will be poor, less likely that fibre and micronutrient intake will be chronically low, and less likely that the diet will be dominated by foods that provide calories without much structural nutritional value.

This becomes increasingly relevant with age because muscle loss rarely happens for one reason alone. It usually develops in the context of multiple pressures: lower activity, reduced appetite, inconsistent protein intake, illness, inflammation, weight fluctuations, and poorer overall diet quality. A stronger dietary pattern may not solve all of those problems by itself, but it can reduce the nutritional instability that allows them to compound.

The Mediterranean-style pattern is often discussed in healthy ageing research for exactly this reason. It is not simply associated with one narrow outcome. It is repeatedly linked with broader markers of resilience, function, and chronic disease risk. That broader association matters in a book like this because muscle preservation is not only about muscle tissue in isolation. It is about preserving strength, movement, recovery, and independence within the full context of ageing.

Not a Prescription, but a Model

It is important not to turn Mediterranean-style eating into a rigid prescription. Many readers will not eat Mediterranean foods in any traditional sense, and they do not need to. The value of this pattern lies in its principles, not in copying a regional menu. A person can eat within very different cultural food traditions and still follow the same muscle-supportive logic: minimally processed staples, regular protein-containing foods, plant variety, better fat quality, and fewer foods that displace nourishment.

That distinction matters because readers often assume that evidence for one dietary pattern means they must adopt it literally. In reality, the lesson is broader. The best-supported dietary patterns for muscle preservation are not successful because they are trendy or romanticised. They are successful because they are nutritionally organised. They make good eating more likely on an ordinary Tuesday, not just in theory.

In Practical Terms

In practical terms, readers do not need to "go Mediterranean" in a performative way. They need to ask whether their current pattern reflects the same general strengths. Does it include enough protein-containing foods across the day? Does it include legumes, vegetables, fruit, and other fibre-rich staples regularly? Is most of the diet built from recognisable foods, or from industrially formulated convenience products? Are meals constructed around nourishment, or around whatever is easiest in the moment?

In practical terms, this section is less about naming the ideal diet and more about identifying the traits that keep showing up in the research. High-quality eating patterns support muscle because they improve the overall odds of adequacy, consistency, and long-term adherence. That is their real strength.

Ultra-Processed Foods and the Erosion of Diet Quality

Ultra-processed foods are now a major part of modern eating patterns, and that matters for muscle preservation not because every packaged food is harmful, but because a diet built heavily around these products often becomes nutritionally weaker over time. These foods are typically designed for convenience, hyper-palatability, long shelf life, and repeated consumption. They can make eating easy, but they do not always make nourishment easy.

From a muscle-health perspective, the problem is rarely one single ingredient. The bigger issue is dietary displacement. When ultra-processed foods take over the pattern, they often crowd out foods that are more useful for maintaining muscle and supporting healthy ageing. Meals become less anchored around meaningful protein sources, fibre intake often drops, diet quality tends to narrow, and overall eating can become more energy-dense without becoming more nutritionally supportive.

This is one reason the conversation around ultra-processed foods needs to stay practical. The goal is not to create fear around every item in a wrapper. The concern is what happens when these foods stop being occasional helpers and become the default structure of the diet.

Why They Can Work Against Muscle Preservation

A muscle-preserving diet depends on nutritional reliability. It works best when the day regularly delivers enough protein, enough total food, and a broad enough range of whole or minimally processed foods to support overall health. Heavy reliance on ultra-processed foods can interfere with that in several ways.

First, these diets are often less effective at supporting consistent protein adequacy across the day. A person may consume plenty of calories while still eating too little high-quality protein at breakfast or lunch, or too little protein overall. Second, ultra-processed dietary patterns often bring lower fibre and poorer overall diet quality, which tends to reflect a weaker nutritional environment more broadly. Third, these patterns may encourage passive overconsumption of energy while still leaving important nutritional needs under-met.

This creates an important distinction. A diet can be energy-rich and still be muscle-poor. That is particularly relevant in midlife and older age, where excess body weight does not automatically protect against low muscle mass, declining strength, or poor muscle quality. In practical terms, a person can be eating more than enough while still eating in a way that does not preserve muscle well.

Association, Not Oversimplification

The evidence linking ultra-processed food intake with frailty and sarcopenia-related outcomes is growing, but it should be discussed carefully. This is not an area where every finding is identical, and it would be too strong to say that ultra-processed foods directly cause muscle loss in a simple one-to-one way. What the research more reasonably suggests is that high intake of these foods often tracks with poorer ageing-related outcomes, including patterns that are less supportive of muscle health.

That nuance matters. It keeps the argument credible. The point is not that one protein bar, frozen meal, or packaged yoghurt is a problem. The point is that when a large share of the diet is made up of industrially formulated foods that displace more nourishing staples, the overall pattern tends to move in the wrong direction.

In that sense, ultra-processed foods are best understood as part of a bigger dietary story. They often signal a pattern that is lower in food quality, lower in structural nourishment, and less supportive of long-term physical resilience.

What This Looks Like in Real Life

In real life, erosion of diet quality usually happens gradually. It may begin with convenience replacing meal structure. Breakfast becomes a pastry or nothing at all. Lunch becomes snack foods, takeaway, or something eaten on the run. Dinner may still look substantial, but the day as a whole has become thin in the areas that matter most. Protein is inconsistent, fibre is low, and much of the intake is coming from products designed more for convenience and reward than for nourishment.

This pattern is common because it fits modern life. It suits busy schedules, low energy, limited cooking skills, and aggressive food marketing. That makes it understandable, but not neutral. Over time, a diet built this way can make muscle-preserving nutrition harder to achieve without the person even realising it.

Older adults can be especially vulnerable here, though for different reasons. Some may rely more heavily on convenience foods because of fatigue, reduced mobility, bereavement, or limited appetite. Others may eat less overall and choose foods that are easy to consume but not especially nutrient-dense. In both cases, the result can be the same: the diet becomes easier to eat, but less effective at preserving muscle.

Reducing Dependence Without Becoming Extreme

A useful response is not to ban ultra-processed foods altogether. That would be unrealistic for most people and unnecessary for the purposes of this book. A better approach is to reduce dependence on them as the dietary backbone. Some convenience foods can still fit within a strong overall pattern, especially when they help maintain adequate intake during busy or low-capacity periods. The issue is whether they are supporting a good structure or replacing it.

This is where many people get stuck in all-or-nothing thinking. They assume that if some packaged foods remain in the diet, they have failed. In reality, the more practical goal is to improve the ratio. The stronger the diet becomes in whole or minimally processed staples, the less damage convenience foods tend to do to the pattern overall.

That means the question is not, "Do I ever eat ultra-processed foods?" The more useful question is, "What proportion of my usual diet depends on them?" If most meals are built from packaged snack items, refined takeaway foods, sugary drinks, confectionery, or heavily processed ready-made products, then the diet pattern is likely working against muscle preservation. If these foods appear occasionally within a broader, higher-quality pattern, that is a very different situation.

In Practical Terms

In practical terms, many people do not need a dramatic dietary overhaul. They need to strengthen the nutritional centre of the diet. That means making sure real meals remain the norm, not the exception. It means anchoring the day with more meaningful protein sources and more fibre-rich foods, and using convenience products more selectively.

In practical terms, one of the clearest warning signs is when meals stop looking like meals. Grazing on snack foods, relying on takeaway several times a week, skipping meals and then overeating processed foods later in the day, or treating highly packaged products as the main source of nourishment are all signs that diet quality may be eroding.

In practical terms, the aim is not food purity. It is dietary direction. A muscle-preserving pattern becomes easier to maintain when the bulk of the diet is built from foods that genuinely contribute to nourishment, and when ultra-processed foods play a smaller supporting role rather than becoming the foundation.

Protein Distribution Within Real Dietary Patterns

Protein intake is often discussed as a daily total, and that is certainly important, but total intake is only part of the picture. In real life, the way protein is distributed across the day also matters. Many adults do not eat too little protein because they are intentionally avoiding it. They fall short because their eating pattern makes adequate protein inconsistent. Breakfast may contain very little protein, lunch may be light or skipped, and most protein may be left to the evening meal. On paper, that can still look like a normal day of eating. In practice, it may be a weaker pattern for preserving muscle.

This becomes more relevant with age. Older adults often need a stronger nutritional signal from meals to support muscle maintenance effectively. When protein intake is repeatedly clustered into one meal, the overall pattern may be less supportive than one in which each main meal contributes meaningfully. This does not mean every meal must be identical, nor does it mean people need to count grams obsessively from morning to night. It means that a more even pattern is often a more useful one.

A muscle-preserving diet, then, is not only about eating enough protein eventually. It is about creating a rhythm of intake that gives the body repeated opportunities to use it well.

The Common Real-World Pattern

In many Western-style diets, protein is heavily skewed toward dinner. Breakfast is often built around toast, cereal, fruit, or coffee. Lunch may be rushed, snack-based, or nutritionally thin. Dinner then carries most of the day's meaningful protein. This pattern is easy to fall into because it fits work schedules, family routines, and appetite habits, but it creates a nutritional imbalance across the day.

That imbalance matters because protein distribution is not just a technical sports nutrition issue. It is a practical ageing issue. If breakfast and lunch contribute very little, then the entire day depends on one meal to do too much. For younger adults with strong appetites and robust muscle responsiveness, this may be less of a problem. For older adults, it is a riskier strategy. Appetite may be reduced, meal size tolerance may be lower, and illness or fatigue may make large evening meals less reliable.

In other words, uneven distribution is not always a problem because dinner is bad. It is a problem because the rest of the day may be doing too little.

Distribution Supports Pattern Quality

One of the most useful things about thinking in terms of protein distribution is that it improves the whole dietary pattern, not just protein intake in isolation. Once a person starts asking whether each main meal contains a real protein source, meals often become more structured overall. Breakfast becomes more substantial. Lunch becomes less likely to be skipped or replaced by snack foods. The day begins to look more like a series of proper meals and less like a drift toward a single large dinner.

This is one reason protein distribution belongs in a chapter about dietary patterns rather than only in a protein chapter. It helps shape the architecture of the day. It pushes eating away from nutritional randomness and toward greater consistency. That, in turn, makes muscle-preserving nutrition easier to maintain without turning the diet into a rigid protocol.

It also helps reinforce another important point: protein does not need to come from one type of food. A more evenly distributed pattern can be built with dairy foods, eggs, fish, meat, legumes, soy foods, or other protein-containing staples. The key issue is not ideology. It is whether the diet repeatedly delivers enough meaningful protein across the day in a way that is realistic and sustainable.

Why Dinner Alone Is Not Enough

Many people assume that a high-protein dinner can compensate for a low-protein day. To some extent it may help, but it is not the strongest pattern to rely on long term. Muscle preservation is generally better served by repeated adequate meals than by one large nutritional correction at the end of the day.

This is particularly important in older age, when appetite and eating capacity often become less predictable. A person may plan to "catch up" at dinner and then find they are tired, unwell, busy, or simply not hungry enough to eat the amount they expected. When too much of the day's nutrition depends on that one moment, the pattern becomes fragile.

A stronger approach is to reduce the need for compensation in the first place. If breakfast, lunch, and dinner all make a meaningful contribution, the day becomes more resilient. Even if one meal is smaller than usual, the pattern still holds.

What Better Distribution Looks Like in Practice

Better protein distribution does not require perfectly equal meals. It simply means avoiding the extreme pattern in which one meal carries nearly all the nutritional weight. Most people will do well when each main meal contains a recognisable protein anchor. That anchor may vary from meal to meal and from person to person, but the principle is the same: breakfast should count, lunch should count, and dinner should not have to rescue the day.

This is often a more useful and realistic message than giving people abstract protein maths. Many readers do not need a formula first. They need a practical lens. When looking at a meal, the question becomes simple: does this meal contain enough real protein to meaningfully contribute to the day, or is it mostly built from refined carbohydrates, snack foods, or convenience items with little substance behind them?

That shift in thinking can be powerful because it changes behaviour without making eating feel clinical. A person does not need to become perfect. They need to stop allowing the day to become protein-light until evening.

In Practical Terms

In practical terms, breakfast is often the best place to improve distribution because it is where many adults fall shortest. A breakfast that contains almost no protein may be convenient, but repeated over time it leaves the day nutritionally back-loaded. Simply strengthening the first meal can make the rest of the day easier.

In practical terms, lunch matters just as much. A skipped lunch, a pastry, or a handful of snack foods may get someone through a busy afternoon, but it does little to support a muscle-preserving pattern. A more structured lunch helps spread protein intake more effectively and reduces the pressure on dinner to compensate.

In practical terms, the goal is not precision for its own sake. It is better patterning. When protein is distributed more sensibly across the day, the entire diet usually becomes more stable, more nourishing, and more supportive of healthy ageing.

Fibre, Whole Foods, and Their Role in Muscle Health

Fibre is not usually the first nutrient people think about when discussing muscle preservation. Protein understandably receives most of the attention, because it directly supports muscle protein synthesis and tissue repair. Yet, as discussed earlier in this book, muscle health is shaped by the broader nutritional environment in which protein is consumed, not by protein alone. Fibre belongs in this conversation because higher-fibre diets tend to reflect stronger overall dietary patterns, and stronger dietary patterns are more consistently associated with better ageing outcomes.

This is an important distinction. Fibre is not being presented here as a direct substitute for protein, nor as a single nutrient that can preserve muscle on its own. Its value lies in what it often represents. Diets rich in fibre tend to include more legumes, vegetables, fruit, and whole grains, and those foods usually arrive as part of a broader pattern that is less dependent on ultra-processed products and more supportive of nutritional adequacy. In that sense, fibre is often a marker of a better-organised diet.

Fibre as a Marker of Diet Quality

One reason fibre matters in this chapter is that it helps reveal the difference between a diet that is merely sufficient in calories and a diet that is genuinely supportive of long-term function. A person may eat enough food, and even enough protein, while still eating in a way that is narrow, highly processed, and poor in plant-food variety. Over time, that kind of pattern can limit the broader nutritional support that ageing muscle depends on.

Higher-fibre eating patterns tend to be built from foods that bring multiple advantages at once. Legumes, vegetables, fruit, and whole grains do not provide fibre in isolation. They also tend to improve micronutrient intake, carbohydrate quality, meal structure, and overall dietary diversity. As noted earlier in this chapter, muscle-preserving nutrition works best when meals are built around real food anchors rather than scattered convenience intake. Fibre-rich foods often help create exactly that structure.

This is why fibre is useful as a pattern-level concept. It helps shift the conversation away from thinking only in terms of isolated nutrients and toward asking whether the diet as a whole is doing its job well.

The Broader Nutritional Environment

Ageing muscle does not exist in a vacuum. It is influenced by inflammation, metabolic health, appetite, food quality, and long-term dietary consistency. A broader nutritional environment that includes regular whole foods is more likely to support those systems than one dominated by refined, heavily processed foods. This does not mean every whole food is automatically beneficial or that every processed food is harmful. It means the overall direction of the diet matters.

Whole-food patterns tend to create a steadier nutritional base. Meals are more likely to contain a meaningful combination of protein, plant foods, and energy, rather than being driven mainly by convenience and hyper-palatability. This matters because muscle preservation is often undermined not by dramatic errors, but by repeated small deficits in dietary quality. A breakfast with little substance, a skipped lunch, a snack-based afternoon, and a processed dinner may not feel extreme in the moment, but repeated across years it creates a weaker nutritional environment for preserving muscle.

As discussed earlier in this chapter, the problem is rarely one single food. It is the pattern that forms when better foods are displaced too often by easier, less nourishing options. Fibre-rich whole foods help counter that drift by making the pattern more substantial, more diverse, and more nutritionally reliable.

Why Whole-Food Quality Matters More With Age

In younger adults, the body can often tolerate a fair amount of nutritional inconsistency without obvious consequences. In midlife and older age, the margin for error becomes smaller. Appetite may decline, anabolic responsiveness may be reduced, and recovery may become more sensitive to gaps in diet quality. Under those conditions, the broader nutritional environment matters more, not less.

This is one reason fibre-rich whole foods deserve attention. They tend to improve the background quality of the diet without requiring extreme restriction or complicated rules. They support a pattern in which meals are more likely to be balanced, more likely to include useful plant foods, and less likely to rely heavily on ultra-processed items. That does not make fibre a magic ingredient. It makes it part of a more supportive setting for healthy ageing.

There is also a practical point here. When whole foods are regularly present, people are often less dependent on packaged products to construct meals. That usually improves consistency, which is one of the central themes of this book. Muscle-preserving nutrition is not built from occasional ideal meals. It is built from a dietary pattern that is good enough, often enough, for long enough.

Whole Foods Without Idealism

It is easy for discussions of whole foods to drift into unrealistic purity. That is not the intention here. Whole-food emphasis does not mean every meal must be rustic, home-cooked, or free from convenience. It means the centre of the diet should be built from foods that still resemble their original ingredients often enough to create a stronger nutritional base.

This matters because most people do not fail through lack of knowledge. They fail through lack of sustainability. If a whole-food approach is framed too rigidly, it becomes fragile and often collapses under normal life pressure. A more useful approach is to treat whole foods as the backbone of the diet and allow practical flexibility around that backbone.

As discussed earlier in this chapter, a durable dietary pattern is more useful than a perfect one. Whole foods support muscle preservation best when they are regular and repeatable, not when they are treated as part of an all-or-nothing identity.

In Practical Terms

In practical terms, this section is not telling readers to chase fibre for its own sake. It is encouraging them to look at whether fibre-rich whole foods are showing up often enough to indicate a stronger overall pattern. If meals rarely include legumes, vegetables, fruit, or whole grains, that usually signals a broader dietary weakness, not simply a low fibre intake.

In practical terms, one of the simplest ways to improve the broader nutritional environment is to stop building meals around what is fastest and start building them around what makes the pattern sturdier. That may mean making sure plant foods are present more often, making meals look more like meals, and relying less on refined convenience intake as the default.

In practical terms, the aim is not to turn the chapter into a gut-health manifesto or a clean-eating lecture. The point is simpler than that. A diet that regularly includes fibre-rich whole foods is usually a diet that is better organised for long-term muscle preservation, because it is more likely to support adequacy, consistency, and overall nutritional stability.

Putting the Dietary Pattern Together Across Midlife and Older Age

By this point in the chapter, the central message should be clear: muscle-preserving nutrition is not built from one perfect food, one perfect diet name, or one flawless week of eating. It is built from the repeated structure of your diet over time. As discussed earlier in this chapter, the strongest dietary patterns tend to make a few things easier at once. They help you eat enough protein, reduce overreliance on ultra-processed foods, include fibre-rich whole foods regularly, and create enough nutritional consistency to support muscle maintenance across the years.

This is why the most useful question is not, "What is the best diet?" The more useful question is, "Does my current pattern reliably support my muscle health?" That shift matters because it moves your focus away from diet labels and toward what your way of eating is actually doing. A dietary pattern is only helpful if it works in real life and still gives your muscles the support they depend on.

Midlife as a Turning Point

Midlife is often the stage when your nutritional habits begin to matter more visibly. You may still have a reasonable amount of muscle, but recovery is often less forgiving, body composition may begin to shift more easily, and long periods of inconsistency can leave a clearer mark. This does not mean muscle decline suddenly begins in midlife, but it is often the point at which your earlier habits either start to protect your function or begin to expose weaknesses in your routine.

This is also when you may become vulnerable to a mismatch between intention and reality. You may feel that you are still eating "normally," yet your pattern may now include frequent meal skipping, low-protein breakfasts, high convenience intake, or repeated periods of under-fuelling during stressful weeks. In younger adulthood, you may have tolerated this more easily. In midlife, those same habits can carry more consequence.

For that reason, midlife is less a crisis point than a correction point. It is the stage where tightening the structure of your diet can have a meaningful long-term return. A more consistent protein pattern, better meal quality, and less drift toward convenience-dominated eating can all help protect the reserve that becomes increasingly valuable later on.

Older Age and a Smaller Margin for Error

In older age, the same general dietary principles still apply, but their importance becomes sharper. Your appetite may decline, your meals may become smaller, illness may interrupt your routine more often, and your muscle may respond less strongly to nutritional signals. As noted earlier in this book, these changes do not make muscle preservation impossible, but they do make the system less forgiving.

This is why dietary patterns that may seem only moderately important in midlife can become highly important in later decades. If you skip meals, rely heavily on low protein convenience foods, or eat very little through the day, you may not simply be eating lightly. You may be eating in a way that steadily works against muscle maintenance, especially if your activity levels are also falling.

At the same time, older age is exactly when rigid nutritional rules become less useful. Your eating pattern still needs to be practical. It has to work with changing appetite, energy, health, and routine. At this stage of life, the goal is usually not dietary perfection. It is preserving your function, your independence, and your resilience under real-world conditions.

Different Stages, Same Core Structure

Although midlife and older age bring different challenges, the underlying pattern remains remarkably similar. In both stages, the goal is to build meals around meaningful protein, maintain enough total intake to support your body, include fibre-rich whole foods regularly, and avoid letting ultra-processed foods become the backbone of your diet. What changes is the level of attention required.

In midlife, this pattern is often about prevention and reserve-building. In older age, it becomes more directly protective. But the structure itself does not need to be reinvented. This is one of the reassuring features of muscle-preserving nutrition: you do not need a completely different system for every decade of life. You need the same basic pattern, applied with greater care as physiological vulnerability increases.

That continuity matters because it makes the strategy more sustainable. You do not need to learn an entirely new way of eating every time life changes. You need to understand which parts of the pattern become more important, and why.

When the Pattern Breaks Down

One of the most practical ways to understand a muscle-preserving diet is to recognise what usually causes it to fail. In most cases, the breakdown is gradual rather than dramatic. Your meals become less structured. Protein becomes inconsistent. Convenience foods begin to replace real meals. Your appetite drops, but your pattern is not adjusted to compensate. Stress, illness, or time pressure push your diet into survival mode, and what was meant to be temporary becomes normal.

This matters because it reminds you that muscle-preserving nutrition is not usually lost through one indulgent weekend or one poor food choice. It is lost through repeated drift. As discussed earlier in this chapter, the issue is not whether every choice is ideal. It is whether your broader pattern keeps moving in a muscle-supportive direction or slowly erodes without you noticing.

Understanding that drift helps make the solution feel more achievable. In most cases, you do not need a complete nutritional overhaul. You need to restore the structure that has weakened.

In Practical Terms

In practical terms, if you are in midlife, it helps to think in terms of preserving reserve before it becomes urgent. That means paying attention to whether your meals contain enough protein, whether your diet quality is strong more often than not, and whether your week has enough structure to stop you from sliding into nutritionally thin routines.

In practical terms, if you are older, it helps to think in terms of protection and reliability. The goal is not perfection. The goal is making sure your body receives enough nutritional support often enough to maintain function. That may mean using simpler meals, more repeated staples, or convenient protein options when your appetite is low, so long as the overall pattern remains supportive.

In practical terms, the best diet pattern is the one you can live with and repeat. If your structure is steady, flexible, and realistic, it is far more likely to preserve your strength and independence than a pattern that sounds impressive in theory but collapses under pressure.

Conclusion

If you want to preserve muscle across the lifespan, you need more than isolated "good" foods or occasional healthy meals. You need a dietary pattern that repeatedly supports the conditions your muscles depend on. As this chapter has shown, that pattern is not defined by perfection. It is defined by consistency. It helps you eat enough protein, distribute that protein more effectively across the day, include fibre-rich whole foods regularly, and reduce the extent to which ultra-processed foods dominate your usual intake.

One of the most important ideas in this chapter is that your muscles are influenced by the broader nutritional environment, not just by one nutrient in isolation. Protein still matters deeply, but it works best within a pattern that is stable, nourishing, and sustainable. A high-quality dietary pattern makes it easier for you to meet your needs repeatedly, not just occasionally. It supports the kind of long-term structure that becomes increasingly important as appetite, recovery, and metabolic resilience change with age.

This is also why the chapter has focused on dietary patterns rather than rigid food rules. You do not need a perfect diet label. You need a way of eating that works in real life and still gives your muscles enough support to remain functional. As discussed earlier in this chapter, Mediterranean-style and other high-quality eating patterns are useful not because they are fashionable, but because they tend to bring together the features that muscle-preserving nutrition depends on. In contrast, when ultra-processed foods become the backbone of your intake, diet quality often begins to erode in ways that are easy to miss until they become habitual.

Another key message is that muscle-preserving nutrition should change in emphasis as you move through life, even if its core structure stays largely the same. In midlife, a stronger dietary pattern helps you protect reserve before loss becomes more obvious. In older age, that same pattern becomes more directly protective, helping you preserve strength, function, and resilience when the margin for error is smaller. The pattern does not need to become extreme. It needs to become dependable.

If there is a practical takeaway from this chapter, it is this: your usual way of eating matters more than your occasional best efforts. Muscle is preserved through repeated support, not nutritional heroics. When your meals are built around meaningful protein, real food anchors, and a pattern you can sustain, you create a stronger foundation for long-term function.

The next chapter builds on this idea by turning to another major influence on muscle preservation: recovery biology. Because even with good training and a strong diet, your muscles still depend on sleep, stress regulation, and hormonal signals to recover and adapt well across time.

Chapter 8: Recovery Biology: Sleep, Stress, Cortisol, and Growth Hormone

Introduction

If resistance training gives your muscles a reason to stay, recovery biology determines how well your body can respond to that demand. You do not adapt during the workout itself. You adapt afterward, when the body repairs tissue, restores energy balance, regulates inflammation, and decides whether the stress you imposed should be translated into greater strength, better function, or no meaningful change at all. This is why muscle preservation is never just a training question. It is also a recovery question.

In earlier chapters, you have already seen that muscle retention depends on repeated alignment between mechanical stimulus and nutritional support. This chapter adds another layer: the internal conditions that make recovery possible. Sleep quality, stress physiology, cortisol rhythm, growth hormone secretion, and chronic low-grade inflammation all influence whether your body stays in a state that supports repair and adaptation or drifts toward one that gradually erodes muscle and function. These influences matter at every age, but they become more important from midlife onward, when recovery is often less forgiving and the margin for error becomes smaller.

This chapter is not about turning sleep or stress into vague lifestyle slogans. It is about understanding how recovery biology shapes the fate of muscle tissue. If you sleep poorly, live under chronic stress, or remain in a state of persistent low-grade inflammation, your muscles do not experience that as background noise. They experience it as a changed biological environment. Over time, that environment influences muscle retention, training adaptation, appetite regulation, and resilience during periods of illness, interruption, or ageing.

Sleep as a Recovery Signal

Sleep is often treated as a passive state, but for your muscles it functions as an active recovery signal. Good sleep supports the coordination of hormonal rhythms, tissue repair processes, protein turnover, and nervous system recovery. Poor sleep does the opposite. It does not simply leave you tired the next day. It changes the biological setting in which your body tries to maintain and repair muscle.

At the population level, the relationship between sleep and sarcopenia is now difficult to ignore. Research consistently shows that abnormal sleep duration, especially short sleep, is associated with a higher likelihood of sarcopenia-related outcomes, and poor sleep quality is also linked with weaker muscle-related health in older adults. The relationship is not perfectly linear, and it would be too simplistic to say that every extra hour of sleep is always better. But the broader message is clear. When sleep is regularly poor, muscle health tends to suffer.

This matters because sleep loss rarely arrives in isolation. It usually travels with other pressures that compound its effects: higher perceived stress, poorer food choices, lower training quality, reduced motivation to move, and more erratic recovery patterns. Over time, that combination can shift you into a state where muscle is no longer being supported as reliably as you think. You may still be exercising and eating reasonably well, yet if sleep is chronically disrupted, the body is recovering in a less favourable environment.

This is particularly important from midlife onward. As you age, sleep architecture changes. Deep sleep often declines, awakenings can become more frequent, and total sleep may feel less restorative even when time in bed appears adequate. That means the quality of recovery can deteriorate quietly over time. If you do not recognise that shift, it is easy to attribute slower progress, poorer recovery, and changes in body composition only to ageing itself, when sleep disruption may be part of the process driving those changes.

Why Sleep Changes Muscle Biology

Sleep matters for muscle not only because it makes you feel better, but because it changes protein metabolism and the hormonal environment that governs tissue maintenance. Human research has shown that even a single night of total sleep deprivation can reduce muscle protein synthesis and shift the hormonal environment in a more catabolic direction. That matters because it shows that sleep is not merely associated with muscle outcomes from a distance. It can directly influence the biological processes that determine whether muscle is being maintained or not.

This helps explain why repeated poor sleep becomes more significant over time. Muscle protein synthesis is not a once-a-week event. It is part of an ongoing turnover process, and your long-term muscle status reflects the cumulative outcome of repeated days and nights of signalling. If sleep repeatedly undermines that process, the result may not be obvious overnight, but over months and years it can contribute to measurable decline.

Sleep restriction also affects how well you recover from exercise. Research examining sleep deprivation and muscle recovery after exercise-induced damage suggests that poor sleep can alter inflammatory and hormonal responses even when overt performance recovery is not always dramatically impaired in the short term. In other words, you may still be able to train while under-recovered, but that does not mean recovery biology is functioning optimally beneath the surface. Many adults judge recovery only by whether they can push through a session, not by whether the body is actually adapting well.

As discussed earlier in this book, muscle preservation depends on repeated, reliable support. Sleep contributes to that reliability by helping maintain a more anabolic environment, restoring nervous system readiness, and reducing the degree to which stress physiology remains elevated across the day. When sleep quality falls, that whole support system becomes less stable. Your muscles are still trying to repair and adapt, but they are doing so in a less favourable setting.

This is one reason sleep should be understood as part of muscle strategy rather than as a separate wellness topic. If you are training hard, eating well, and still recovering poorly, sleep is often one of the first places where the biological explanation begins.

Stress Physiology, Cortisol, and Muscle Retention

Stress is not inherently harmful. Acute stress responses are part of normal physiology. They help you mobilise energy, increase alertness, and respond to challenge. The problem begins when stress is no longer brief and adaptive, but persistent and poorly resolved. When that happens, the endocrine system begins to shift in ways that can work against muscle preservation.

Cortisol sits at the centre of this discussion. It is often reduced to a caricature in popular health culture, but in reality it is a necessary hormone involved in energy regulation, immune balance, and stress adaptation. The issue is not that cortisol exists. The issue is what happens when cortisol remains elevated too often, when its rhythm becomes dysregulated, or when the body is repeatedly driven into a state where catabolic signalling is chronically favoured over recovery. Chronic activation of the stress system influences metabolism, immune function, and tissue maintenance in ways that are highly relevant to muscle.

The link between cortisol and muscle is stronger than vague theory. Evidence supports the view that higher cortisol exposure is associated with reductions in muscle strength and lean mass, and newer work strengthens the case that chronic stress can promote skeletal muscle atrophy through multiple pathways, including altered protein turnover, impaired anabolic signalling, and changes in glucose handling.

This is especially relevant in midlife and older age because stress physiology changes with age. Adrenal responsiveness, cortisol rhythm, sleep quality, metabolic flexibility, and inflammatory tone all shift over time. That means chronic stress may not affect a 65-year-old body in exactly the same way it affects a 25-year-old one. In later decades, stress often arrives on top of reduced sleep quality, lower activity, higher caregiving burden, illness, pain, or metabolic dysfunction. Under those conditions, cortisol is not acting alone. It becomes part of a broader recovery-disruptive environment.

In practical terms, chronic stress can work against your muscle in two ways at once. First, it alters the biology of recovery, making the internal environment less supportive of repair and adaptation. Second, it changes behaviour. It disrupts sleep, shifts appetite, reduces motivation to train, increases reliance on convenience foods, and makes consistency harder to maintain. Over time, those biological and behavioural effects reinforce each other.

As noted earlier in this book, muscle decline is rarely caused by one single factor. Chronic stress is a good example of that principle. It does not usually destroy muscle in one dramatic event. It works more quietly by reshaping the environment in which your muscles are trying to survive, recover, and adapt.

Growth Hormone, Slow-Wave Sleep, and Ageing

Growth hormone has been heavily mythologised, but its real role in this chapter is more specific and more useful. It matters because it helps illustrate that sleep is not just rest. Sleep is a period of coordinated endocrine activity, and one of the most reproducible hormonal events in healthy adults is the major pulse of growth hormone that occurs shortly after sleep onset, especially in association with slow-wave sleep.

This relationship has been established for decades. Sleep physiology research has shown that growth hormone secretion is tightly linked to slow-wave sleep, and later work clarified that ageing is associated with reductions in both slow-wave sleep and nocturnal growth hormone secretion. In simple terms, the decline in deep sleep that often occurs with age is not just a sleep-quality issue. It also reflects a change in the endocrine pattern associated with recovery and tissue maintenance.

That does not mean growth hormone is a magic key to youthful muscle. It is more accurate to say that growth hormone is one part of a broader anabolic environment, and that environment becomes less robust with age. Clinical reviews of growth hormone and ageing note that age-related reductions in growth hormone are associated with changes in body composition, including reduced lean mass and increased adiposity. But this is not a chapter about hormone replacement. It is a chapter about how normal ageing sleep biology influences the internal environment in which muscle is maintained.

Cortisol belongs in this section too, because sleep architecture influences more than one hormonal rhythm. Research in older adults has shown that disturbed sleep can be associated with altered daytime cortisol patterns, while longer and better sleep can buffer some of the age-related rise in diurnal cortisol. This matters because growth hormone and cortisol are moving in opposite directions from a recovery standpoint. More consolidated sleep supports a more favourable anabolic pattern, while poor sleep can push the system toward one that is more catabolic and less restorative.

For you, the practical meaning is straightforward. Sleep is not valuable only because you feel sharper the next day. It is valuable because it helps preserve the hormonal timing that supports recovery. As you age, that timing becomes easier to disrupt and harder to restore casually. That is one reason sleep quality becomes more important, not less, with advancing age.

As discussed earlier in this chapter, muscle preservation depends on more than food and training. Growth hormone physiology makes that point very clearly. The body recovers within a hormonal rhythm, and that rhythm is strongly shaped by sleep.

Inflammaging and Blunted Adaptation

Inflammation is an essential biological process, but like stress, it becomes harmful when it remains chronically elevated at low levels for long periods. In ageing biology, this persistent background inflammation is often referred to as inflammaging. It does not usually look dramatic. It is not the same as acute infection or obvious illness. Instead, it reflects a long-term shift toward a more inflammatory internal state, and that state has important consequences for muscle retention and adaptation.

Research on inflammaging and sarcopenia describes this low-grade inflammatory environment as one of the core contributors to age-related muscle decline. Pro-inflammatory cytokines can interfere with anabolic signalling, promote protein breakdown pathways, alter mitochondrial function, and reduce the efficiency with which aged muscle responds to exercise and nutrition. This is one reason ageing muscle may seem less responsive even when training and diet are present. The issue is not always lack of effort. Sometimes the biological environment itself has become less cooperative.

This also helps explain why this is a chapter about recovery biology rather than simply sleep and stress. Chronic low-grade inflammation is part of the same story. It changes how well you recover, how effectively you adapt, and how strongly your body responds to the same training stimulus that once produced better results. Recent work specifically linking age-associated inflammation to skeletal muscle health and exercise adaptation supports the idea that inflammation can blunt the response to training, not just contribute to passive decline.

The causes of inflammaging are multiple. Age-related immune change, increased visceral adiposity, inactivity, poor sleep, chronic stress, metabolic dysfunction, and persistent low-grade disease burden all contribute. Poor sleep can worsen inflammatory tone. Chronic stress can worsen inflammatory tone. Excess adiposity can worsen inflammatory tone. Together, they can create a self-reinforcing cycle that makes muscle preservation harder.

Importantly, inflammation should not be described as an irreversible fate. It is influenced by behaviour and environment. Exercise, body composition improvement, better sleep, reduced stress load, and stronger diet quality can all help make the inflammatory environment less hostile to muscle. This does not mean inflammation disappears. It means the background conditions become more favourable for recovery and adaptation.

As discussed earlier in this book, muscle ageing is not driven by a single mechanism. Inflammaging is a powerful example of that. It sits at the intersection of immune ageing, metabolic health, stress biology, and physical function. If you want to preserve muscle across time, you cannot afford to think of inflammation as a distant medical issue. It is part of the environment in which your muscles either hold their ground or gradually lose it.

Appetite Regulation Under Poor Sleep and Stress

Recovery biology does not affect muscle only through tissue-level signalling. It also affects how you eat. This matters because appetite regulation is one of the places where sleep, stress, and muscle preservation overlap in very practical ways.

Sleep deprivation alters central appetite regulation and tends to shift eating in a less favourable direction. Reviews and meta-analyses show that inadequate sleep can increase desire to eat, affect food selection, and change overall intake patterns. In practical terms, poor sleep often makes highly rewarding, energy-dense foods more appealing while making routine, structured eating harder to maintain. That does not automatically cause muscle loss, but it can weaken the dietary pattern that supports muscle over time.

Stress affects appetite too, though not always in the same direction. Some people under chronic stress eat more, especially more convenient and energy-dense foods. Others lose appetite and under-eat. Both patterns can be relevant to muscle. Overeating can worsen adiposity and inflammation while still failing to provide a genuinely muscle-supportive pattern. Under-eating can reduce total protein and energy intake, making muscle more vulnerable to negative protein balance. In later life, where appetite may already be reduced, the combination of stress and low intake can be especially problematic.

This is one reason appetite regulation deserves a place in a chapter about recovery. Your muscles depend on food, but food intake depends partly on how sleep and stress are shaping your hunger, satiety, routine, and decision-making. If poor sleep and chronic stress are repeatedly pushing your diet off course, then the nutritional strategy discussed in earlier chapters becomes harder to execute, even if you understand it intellectually.

Older adults bring an additional layer to this issue because ageing itself can change appetite regulation. Appetite often declines in later life, which means the body may need more nutritional intention at exactly the stage when spontaneous intake becomes less reliable. If poor sleep, stress, illness, or inflammation are added to that background, maintaining adequate intake becomes even harder. That matters because, as noted earlier in this book, muscle is easier to preserve than to rebuild after decline.

In practical terms, sleep and stress can influence your muscle-preserving diet in one of two broad ways. They can push you toward overconsumption of low-quality foods, or they can reduce your intake so much that protein and energy adequacy start to slip. Neither pattern is ideal. Both remind you that recovery biology is shaping nutrition behaviour whether you notice it or not.

Bringing Recovery Biology Together

By this point, the pattern should be clear. Sleep, stress, cortisol regulation, growth hormone secretion, inflammation, and appetite are not separate side issues. They are interconnected parts of the environment in which your muscles are trying to survive and adapt.

When recovery biology is working well, sleep is more restorative, cortisol rhythms are more stable, inflammatory tone is lower, appetite is easier to regulate, and the body is more likely to respond productively to training and nutrition. When recovery biology is chronically disturbed, the opposite tends to happen. Sleep becomes fragmented, stress signalling stays elevated, appetite becomes less reliable, inflammation becomes more persistent, and the muscle-preserving effect of good training and sound nutrition becomes harder to realise fully.

This is why some people feel they are doing everything right and still not recovering well. The missing piece is sometimes not another supplement, not another workout, and not another dietary rule. It is the biological environment in which those strategies are being applied. Recovery is not a luxury add-on to muscle preservation. It is one of the conditions that makes muscle preservation possible.

For you, the practical lesson is not that you need perfect sleep or a stress-free life. Neither is realistic. The lesson is that recovery biology deserves deliberate attention because it changes the return you get from everything else you are doing. A good training program works better in a well-recovered body. A strong diet works better in a well-regulated body. If you improve the recovery environment, you often improve the value of the training and nutrition already in place.

Conclusion

Muscle preservation is often described in terms of protein and resistance training, and rightly so. But this chapter has shown that those inputs do not operate in isolation. They are filtered through recovery biology. Sleep quality, stress physiology, cortisol rhythm, growth hormone secretion, chronic low-grade inflammation, and appetite regulation all influence whether your muscles are supported or undermined across time.

One of the most important themes running through this chapter is that poor recovery does not simply make you feel tired. It changes the biological environment in which your muscles are being maintained. Poor sleep is associated with less favourable muscle outcomes and can reduce muscle protein synthesis. Chronic stress and cortisol dysregulation can shift the body toward a more catabolic state. Age-related decline in slow-wave sleep affects the hormonal rhythm linked to growth hormone secretion. Chronic low-grade inflammation can blunt adaptation and promote muscle decline. And sleep and stress together can push your eating pattern in directions that make muscle-supportive nutrition harder to maintain.

This matters even more in midlife and older age, when the margin for error becomes smaller. You can no longer assume that your body will compensate easily for chronic sleep debt, persistent stress, or a long-standing inflammatory load. Those pressures may not produce obvious consequences immediately, but over time they alter recovery, reduce resilience, and make muscle retention less reliable.

The encouraging message is that recovery biology is not fixed. You cannot eliminate ageing, and you cannot eliminate all stress, but you can improve the environment in which your body recovers. Better sleep habits, more deliberate stress management, regular movement, stronger diet quality, and reduced chronic inflammatory load all help create conditions in which muscle is more likely to be preserved.

As discussed earlier in this book, muscle matters because it supports function, resilience, and independence. Recovery biology matters because it helps determine whether that muscle is given the conditions it needs to stay. The next chapters continue building that picture by moving further into the systems and strategies that influence muscle preservation across the lifespan.

Chapter 9: The Gut–Muscle Axis and Inflammation

Introduction

Your muscles do not exist in isolation. They are influenced not only by training and nutrition, but also by the internal environment in which those inputs are processed. One of the most important emerging areas in this discussion is the gut–muscle axis: the relationship between gut health, immune signalling, nutrient handling, and skeletal muscle function. This field has gained attention for good reason, but it also needs to be handled carefully. The current evidence does not support exaggerated claims that the microbiome simply "controls" muscle. What it does support is a more measured idea: the state of your gut may influence how well your body maintains muscle, responds to food, regulates inflammation, and adapts to physical stress.

This matters because muscle preservation is shaped by more than the amount of protein you eat or the number of times you train each week. As discussed earlier in this book, muscle is maintained within a broader physiological setting. If inflammation is chronically elevated, if nutrient absorption is impaired, if metabolic signalling becomes less efficient, or if the body is exposed to repeated immune stress, the environment for muscle maintenance changes. The gut sits at the centre of several of these processes. It helps regulate the interface between what you eat and what your body can actually use. It also influences immune tone, intestinal barrier integrity, microbial metabolite production, and the low-grade inflammatory burden that often increases with age.

This is why the gut–muscle axis has become especially relevant in ageing research. Older adults with sarcopenia often show differences in gut microbial composition compared with those without it, and emerging evidence suggests that these differences may be linked with muscle mass, strength, and physical performance. That does not prove that gut dysbiosis directly causes muscle loss in every case. But it does suggest that the condition of the gut may be one part of the biological terrain in which sarcopenia develops.

The idea becomes even more relevant when you consider how many systems meet in the gut. Diet quality influences the microbiome. The microbiome influences microbial metabolites. Those metabolites may affect inflammation, mitochondrial function, insulin sensitivity, and muscle metabolism. Intestinal barrier dysfunction may allow greater exposure to inflammatory compounds. Chronic low-grade inflammation may then interfere with anabolic signalling and muscle recovery. None of this means the gut is the only driver of muscle ageing. It means the gut may help shape how favourable or unfavourable the internal environment becomes.

That distinction is important because this chapter is not about microbiome hype. It is not here to suggest that one probiotic or one gut-health trend will solve sarcopenia. Instead, the goal is to explain what the gut–muscle axis actually means, what the evidence currently supports, and how gut health may influence muscle through immune, metabolic, and nutritional pathways. Some parts of this field are already supported by meaningful human evidence. Other parts remain promising but preliminary. Both realities need to be held together if this chapter is going to be useful.

In practical terms, this chapter adds depth to a point that has already been building through the book: muscle is not only trained and fed. It is also regulated by the state of the systems around it. The gut is one of those systems. If it is functioning well, it may help support the conditions in which muscle can be preserved. If it is functioning poorly, it may contribute to a more inflammatory, less efficient environment that makes muscle maintenance harder over time.

What the Gut–Muscle Axis Actually Means

The term *gut–muscle axis* refers to the relationship between the condition of your gastrointestinal system and the health of your skeletal muscle. At first glance, those systems may seem far apart. One digests food. The other produces movement and force. But in biological terms, they are closely connected. Your muscles depend on nutrients being broken down, absorbed, transported, and used effectively. They also depend on a relatively stable immune and inflammatory environment. The gut influences both.

At the simplest level, the gut–muscle axis begins with digestion and absorption. If food is not digested and absorbed efficiently, the body has less access to the amino acids, vitamins, minerals, and energy substrates required to maintain and repair muscle. This is the most straightforward connection. But the relationship goes further than nutrient delivery. The gut is also home to a dense and metabolically active microbial community that helps shape the body's internal environment in ways that may affect muscle retention and physical function.

These microbes do not simply exist in the background. They interact with dietary components, produce metabolites, influence intestinal barrier integrity, and affect immune signalling. Some of the most discussed microbial products in this area are short-chain fatty acids, which are generated when gut bacteria ferment dietary fibre. These compounds are of interest because they may influence inflammation, insulin sensitivity, mitochondrial function, and the broader metabolic setting in which muscle is maintained. That does not mean short-chain fatty acids are a direct muscle-building tool. It means they are one of the ways the gut may help shape whether the internal environment is more supportive or less supportive of muscle health.

Another major part of the gut–muscle axis is barrier function. A healthy intestinal barrier helps regulate what passes from the gut into circulation. When that barrier becomes less effective, the body may be exposed to greater amounts of bacterial components that promote immune activation and low-grade inflammation. As discussed earlier in this book, chronic low-grade inflammation is one of the major biological conditions associated with muscle decline. In that sense, the gut may influence muscle not only through what it helps you absorb, but also through what it allows into the system when barrier integrity is compromised.

This is where the gut–muscle axis becomes more than a digestion story. It becomes a regulation story. The gut may influence muscle through inflammation, metabolic signalling, insulin sensitivity, mitochondrial efficiency, and possibly even anabolic responsiveness. None of these pathways should be overstated. The field is still developing, and some mechanisms are supported more strongly than others. But taken together, they help explain why muscle health may be affected by the state of the gut even when a person appears to be eating enough food on paper.

Ageing makes this discussion more relevant because the gut environment often changes with age. Microbial diversity can shift, dietary patterns may narrow, medication use becomes more common, appetite can decline, and chronic disease burden often increases. These changes do not affect everyone equally, but they help explain why the gut–muscle axis is now being studied so closely in older adults and in people with sarcopenia. The question is not whether the microbiome alone determines muscle fate. The question is whether age-related changes in gut health may contribute to a less favourable environment for muscle maintenance and recovery.

A useful way to think about the gut–muscle axis is this: your muscles depend on more than the food you eat. They also depend on what your body can absorb, how your immune system is responding, how much inflammatory burden is present, and whether the metabolic environment is helping or hindering repair. The gut sits near the centre of all of those processes. That is why this axis matters.

In practical terms, the gut–muscle axis should not be understood as a separate health niche. It is part of the broader biological environment in which muscle is either supported or undermined. If your gut health is poor, the effect may not show up only as digestive discomfort. It may also influence how well your body handles nutrients, regulates inflammation, and maintains muscle over time.

Gut Dysbiosis and Sarcopenia

One of the main reasons the gut–muscle axis is now taken seriously is that people with sarcopenia often appear to have a different gut microbial profile from those without it. That does not mean a single "bad" bacterium causes muscle loss, and it does not mean the microbiome alone explains why sarcopenia develops. But it does suggest that gut dysbiosis may be part of the broader biological pattern associated with declining muscle mass, strength, and physical function.

The word dysbiosis simply refers to an unfavourable shift in the gut microbial community. This might involve reduced microbial diversity, altered proportions of bacterial groups, or a microbial environment that is less supportive of metabolic and immune stability. In the context of ageing, this matters because gut microbial balance appears to become less robust in many older adults, particularly when diet quality declines, medication use increases, chronic disease burden rises, or physical function begins to deteriorate. These changes do not prove cause and effect, but they do create the kind of environment in which the gut may become a more important contributor to muscle health.

Systematic reviews and meta-analyses now suggest that older adults with sarcopenia often show measurable differences in gut microbiota compared with non-sarcopenic controls. In some studies, this includes lower microbial diversity. In others, it involves shifts in bacterial genera thought to be relevant to inflammation, fibre fermentation, and metabolic regulation. The exact microbial patterns are not identical across studies, which is important to acknowledge. This is still a heterogeneous field, and the microbiome does not present as one neat universal signature of sarcopenia. But the broader trend is consistent enough to matter: sarcopenia is often associated with a gut environment that looks different from that seen in healthier ageing.

This is an important point because it changes how you think about muscle decline. Sarcopenia is not just a story of underused muscle tissue. It is also a story of the internal environment in which that tissue exists. If the gut microbial ecosystem is altered in a way that promotes inflammation, reduces favourable metabolite production, or weakens nutrient handling, then the body may become less supportive of muscle maintenance even before severe muscle loss is obvious. In that sense, gut dysbiosis may not need to be the original trigger to still be clinically relevant. It may help reinforce the progression of decline once the process is underway.

There is also a practical reason this matters. Sarcopenia tends to develop in real-world settings where multiple systems are already under pressure. Older adults may have poorer sleep, lower activity, reduced appetite, more medications, greater metabolic dysfunction, and higher chronic inflammatory burden. The gut microbiome sits in the middle of many of those influences. So while the microbiome should not be treated as the master controller of muscle, it may act as one of the systems through which these pressures converge.

This is where caution is needed. It would be easy to overinterpret the findings and suggest that dysbiosis is the hidden cause behind all muscle decline. That would be too strong. Most of the evidence in this area remains observational, which means it shows association more clearly than causation. A person with sarcopenia may have an altered microbiome because of poorer diet, reduced mobility, illness, or medication exposure rather than because the microbiome changed first. The relationship is likely bidirectional. Muscle decline may worsen gut health, and gut dysfunction may worsen muscle decline. Both can be true at the same time.

That bidirectional possibility is one of the most useful ways to understand the evidence. As physical function declines, diet quality may worsen, activity may fall, and gut microbial quality may deteriorate. As gut health deteriorates, inflammation and metabolic inefficiency may rise, making muscle preservation harder. This does not produce a simple linear model. It produces a feedback loop, and feedback loops are common in ageing biology.

In practical terms, the significance of gut dysbiosis is not that you need to become obsessed with microbiome testing or microbial labels. It is that muscle health may partly reflect the state of the gut ecosystem in which recovery, nutrient use, and immune balance are occurring. If that ecosystem is less stable, muscle may be maintained less effectively across time.

Inflammation, Intestinal Barrier Function, and Muscle Loss

One of the most important ways the gut may influence muscle is through inflammation. This connection matters because muscle does not decline only from inactivity or inadequate protein. It also declines more easily in a body that remains under chronic low-grade immune stress. As discussed earlier in this book, inflammation is not automatically harmful. It is a necessary part of immune defence and tissue repair. The problem begins when inflammation becomes persistent, poorly resolved, and woven into the background of everyday physiology.

The gut plays a central role in this process because it is one of the main interfaces between the outside world and the internal environment of the body. A healthy intestinal lining helps regulate what passes from the digestive tract into circulation. It allows nutrients to be absorbed while limiting the movement of unwanted microbial products and inflammatory triggers. When this barrier is functioning well, it supports stability. When it becomes compromised, the body may be exposed to a greater inflammatory burden.

This is where intestinal permeability becomes relevant. The term is sometimes oversimplified in popular health culture, but the basic principle is sound: if the gut barrier becomes less effective, microbial components may pass more easily into circulation and stimulate immune activation. That does not mean every digestive symptom reflects a damaged gut barrier, and it does not mean barrier dysfunction is the sole cause of systemic inflammation. But it does mean that the gut can be one source of the chronic low-grade immune activity that makes muscle preservation harder over time.

For muscle, the consequences of this inflammatory environment are significant. Chronic low-grade inflammation can interfere with anabolic signalling, promote protein breakdown pathways, impair insulin sensitivity, and reduce the efficiency with which muscle responds to nutrition and training. In practical terms, your body becomes less cooperative. The same exercise and food intake that once produced a good adaptive response may produce less when the inflammatory background is persistently elevated.

This is one reason the gut–muscle axis is closely tied to ageing biology. In older adults, the inflammatory burden often rises even without obvious acute illness. That increase may be shaped by multiple factors at once, including higher visceral adiposity, lower activity, chronic disease, poorer diet quality, medication use, and altered gut microbial composition. The gut does not need to be the only driver of inflammation to still matter. If it adds to the inflammatory load, it becomes part of the environment in which muscle is either preserved or undermined.

Barrier function also helps explain why gut health should not be viewed only as a digestive issue. A person may not think of bowel habits, fermentation, microbial balance, or intestinal integrity as part of muscle health, yet these processes can influence how much immune stress the body is carrying. Over time, that immune stress may shape recovery, nutrient handling, and tissue maintenance in ways that are highly relevant to sarcopenia and functional decline.

There is also an important feedback loop here. As muscle health worsens, physical activity often declines. As activity declines, metabolic health may worsen, inflammatory tone may rise, and gut health may become less favourable. At the same time, poorer gut function may further increase inflammatory pressure and make muscle retention harder. This is one reason muscle decline in older age rarely follows a single straight line. It often becomes self-reinforcing unless something interrupts the cycle.

This section also helps explain why gut-directed strategies are attracting attention in ageing research. If intestinal barrier function and inflammation are part of the muscle story, then improving gut health could, in theory, help create a more favourable internal environment for muscle maintenance. That possibility is biologically plausible, but it should still be treated carefully. The field is promising, but it is not yet at the point where strong therapeutic claims can be made without qualification.

In practical terms, the most useful takeaway is not that inflammation from the gut is the hidden cause of all muscle loss. It is that muscle is easier to preserve in a body that is not carrying an unnecessary inflammatory burden. The gut may be one of the places where that burden is either contained or amplified. That makes intestinal barrier function and inflammatory regulation relevant to muscle, even if they are not the only influences that matter.

Nutrient Absorption, Protein Utilisation, and Anabolic Responsiveness

One of the most practical ways the gut may influence muscle is through nutrient handling. You do not benefit from what you eat simply because it is on the plate. Food has to be broken down, absorbed, and made available to the tissues that need it. For muscle, that includes amino acids, energy substrates, vitamins, and minerals. If the gut environment is less effective at supporting those processes, the nutritional support available to muscle may be weaker than your food intake alone would suggest.

This is an important point because muscle preservation is often discussed as though intake automatically equals use. In reality, there is a difference between consuming enough protein and being in a physiological state that allows that protein to be used effectively. The gut may influence that difference through digestion, absorption efficiency, microbial metabolism, inflammatory tone, and the overall metabolic setting in which nutrients are processed.

Protein is especially relevant here because, as discussed earlier in this book, muscle maintenance depends heavily on the repeated availability and effective use of amino acids. If gut dysfunction contributes to poorer digestion, altered absorption, or a more inflammatory environment, then the body may become less efficient at translating protein intake into muscle-supportive signalling. This does not mean that the gut "switches off" muscle protein synthesis. It means the internal conditions for using protein well may become less favourable.

This is where anabolic responsiveness enters the discussion. Muscle does not respond to food in a vacuum. Its anabolic response depends on more than protein alone. It is shaped by age, training status, inflammation, insulin sensitivity, energy balance, and the broader physiological environment. The gut may matter because it sits upstream of several of these influences. A less healthy gut environment may contribute to low-grade inflammation, poorer metabolic regulation, and altered microbial metabolite production, all of which could make muscle less responsive to nutritional signals over time.

That possibility becomes more relevant in ageing because older adults already tend to be more vulnerable to anabolic resistance. If the body is less responsive to protein with age, then anything that further weakens nutrient handling or increases inflammatory burden may add to the problem. In that context, gut health is not replacing the protein story. It is modifying the conditions in which the protein story plays out.

The microbiome may also influence protein utilisation more indirectly through its relationship with fermentation, amino acid metabolism, and short-chain fatty acid production. These pathways are still being studied, and the field is not yet mature enough to make strong causal claims. But the broader idea is biologically plausible: if the gut microbial ecosystem affects metabolic efficiency and inflammatory tone, it may also affect how effectively the body responds to the nutrients needed for muscle maintenance.

This helps explain why some people may appear to be eating reasonably well and still not getting the full benefit one might expect. The issue may not always be intake alone. It may be that the environment in which those nutrients are being processed is less supportive of adaptation and tissue maintenance. That does not make the gut the sole explanation, but it does make it one relevant part of the picture.

At the same time, caution matters here. The current evidence does not justify dramatic claims that fixing the microbiome will automatically improve protein utilisation or reverse anabolic resistance. The relationship is more subtle than that. What the evidence supports is a careful conclusion: gut health may influence the efficiency with which nutrients are handled and the degree to which muscle remains responsive to them, particularly in older adults living with sarcopenia, inflammation, or metabolic dysfunction.

In practical terms, this section reinforces a larger theme running through the book. Muscle is not preserved by nutrients in isolation. It is preserved when the body is in a state that can digest, absorb, regulate, and use those nutrients effectively. The gut may influence each of those steps. That makes it a relevant part of the muscle-preservation conversation, even if it is not the whole story.

How Diet Patterns Influence the Gut–Muscle Environment

By this point in the chapter, it should be clear that the gut–muscle axis is not just about microbes in isolation. It is also about the kind of environment your daily diet creates. The foods you eat help shape microbial diversity, fermentation patterns, intestinal barrier function, and inflammatory tone. In that sense, diet patterns are not only feeding you. They are also feeding, suppressing, or reshaping the microbial ecosystem that may influence muscle health over time.

This is one of the reasons Chapter 9 connects naturally with the earlier discussion in Chapter 7. As noted earlier in this book, high-quality dietary patterns tend to support muscle not only because they improve protein adequacy, but because they create a broader internal environment that is more stable and less inflammatory. The gut–muscle axis adds another layer to that idea. A diet pattern rich in fibre-containing plant foods, minimally processed staples, and overall dietary variety may help support a more favourable microbial environment than one dominated by ultra-processed foods and low in fermentable substrates.

Fibre matters here for a different reason than it did in Chapter 7. There, the emphasis was on fibre as a marker of diet quality and a sign of a more supportive overall eating pattern. Here, fibre matters because it provides fermentable material for gut microbes. When that fermentation process is functioning well, it can contribute to the production of short-chain fatty acids and other metabolites that may help support barrier function, immune balance, and metabolic regulation. That does not make fibre a direct muscle-building nutrient, but it does make it part of the environment that may indirectly influence muscle maintenance.

Dietary patterns low in fibre and high in ultra-processed foods may move the gut–muscle environment in the opposite direction. These diets are often associated with lower dietary diversity, poorer microbial support, and a more inflammatory metabolic background. As discussed earlier in the book, ultra-processed dietary patterns may also make it harder to maintain consistent protein quality, micronutrient adequacy, and overall nutritional stability. Through the lens of the gut–muscle axis, that same pattern may also contribute to a less favourable microbiome and a weaker intestinal environment.

This is where the idea of a microbiome-supportive dietary pattern becomes useful, but it needs to be framed carefully. The evidence does suggest that dietary patterns associated with a healthier gut microbial profile tend to be linked with lower sarcopenia prevalence and a more favourable inflammatory environment. But this is still mostly associative evidence. It would be too strong to say that one specific diet pattern definitively improves muscle by "fixing" the gut microbiome. A more honest interpretation is that diets supporting a healthier gut environment may also support some of the physiological conditions in which muscle is better preserved.

The practical significance of this is that muscle-preserving nutrition and gut-supportive nutrition are often not separate strategies. They overlap. A diet rich in vegetables, legumes, whole grains, fruit, and other minimally processed foods is already moving in a direction that supports both. It can provide fibre for fermentation, greater dietary diversity, and a more stable nutritional structure while also making it easier to build meals around meaningful protein. This is one reason whole dietary patterns tend to matter more than isolated supplements or trend-driven "gut health" fixes.

Ageing makes this overlap even more important. In later life, appetite may narrow, food variety may drop, and convenience intake may increase. At the same time, microbial diversity may decline and low-grade inflammation may rise. Under those conditions, the quality of the daily diet becomes even more important. A weaker diet pattern may not only reduce protein and micronutrient adequacy, but may also worsen the gut environment in ways that further undermine muscle maintenance.

This also helps explain why Chapter 9 should not drift into hype. The gut–muscle axis is interesting precisely because it connects systems that were once discussed separately. But the safest and most useful takeaway is not that you need to chase special gut-health products. It is that the same broad dietary habits that support muscle preservation are also likely to support a more favourable gut environment.

In practical terms, this means that if your diet pattern is built around meaningful protein, fibre-rich plant foods, and mostly recognisable foods, you are probably already supporting the gut–muscle environment better than someone relying heavily on ultra-processed, low-fibre, nutritionally thin intake. That does not guarantee perfect gut health or perfect muscle preservation. But it does move the system in a more favourable direction.

Can Gut-Targeted Interventions Help?

Once the gut–muscle axis is introduced, the obvious next question is whether you can improve muscle-related outcomes by targeting the gut directly. This is where the evidence becomes interesting, but also where caution matters most. There is growing research on probiotics, prebiotics, synbiotics, and related strategies in older adults and in people at risk of sarcopenia. Some findings are encouraging. But the field is not yet strong enough to justify confident claims that gut-targeted interventions should be treated as a primary solution for muscle loss.

The main reason for caution is that intervention studies remain mixed. Some trials suggest that probiotic or synbiotic strategies may improve aspects of muscle strength, physical performance, or body composition in older adults. Others show limited or inconsistent effects. This does not mean the idea is wrong. It means the evidence is still developing, and the outcomes are not yet consistent enough to treat these interventions as established therapy in the same way resistance training and adequate protein intake are established.

Part of the difficulty is that gut-targeted interventions are not all the same. Different studies use different strains, combinations, doses, treatment durations, and participant populations. Some include people who are already frail or sarcopenic. Others include older adults who are generally healthy. Some interventions are layered on top of exercise or dietary change, while others are tested more narrowly. This makes the field harder to interpret because positive findings in one context do not automatically transfer to another.

There is also a practical issue of biological variability. The microbiome is not identical from person to person, and neither is the ageing process. A gut-targeted intervention may help one person more than another depending on baseline microbial composition, diet quality, inflammatory burden, medication use, metabolic health, and physical function. That variability is one reason the field can look promising in principle while still remaining inconsistent in practice.

Prebiotics and fibre-related strategies deserve attention for a slightly different reason. Rather than introducing live organisms directly, they aim to support the growth or activity of microbial populations that may be beneficial. This fits well with the broader theme of the chapter because it reinforces the idea that diet patterns may shape the gut environment more sustainably than isolated products alone. Even here, however, the most defensible message is still cautious. Supporting a healthier microbial environment may be useful, but it should not be presented as a guaranteed route to better muscle function.

Post-biotics and other emerging gut-directed therapies are also beginning to attract interest. These approaches are conceptually appealing because they focus on microbial products or downstream effects rather than only on changing microbial populations themselves. But at this stage, they belong more to future directions than to firm clinical recommendations. They help show where the field is going, but not yet what should be presented to the reader as settled practice.

This is one reason it is so important to keep the hierarchy of evidence clear. Gut-targeted interventions may become part of future sarcopenia care, especially if better trials continue to show meaningful effects on strength, physical performance, or muscle-related biomarkers. But at present, they should be viewed as supportive and emerging rather than foundational. The strongest muscle-preservation tools remain the ones already established earlier in this book: resistance training, adequate protein intake, strong overall diet quality, and the reduction of chronic inflammatory burden where possible.

In practical terms, this means you should be cautious about any message suggesting that a probiotic product, a gut powder, or a microbiome trend can replace the basics. At best, these strategies may add support in selected cases. They do not replace the need for a well-structured diet, sufficient protein, physical activity, and recovery. The most useful way to think about gut-targeted interventions right now is as possible adjuncts, not as the centre of the plan.

That is also what makes this area worth watching. The evidence is not strong enough yet for hype, but it is strong enough to justify serious interest. If future research becomes more precise about which interventions help, for whom, and under what conditions, the gut–muscle axis may eventually play a larger role in clinical and practical muscle-preservation strategies. For now, it is best approached with interest, but also with discipline.

Conclusion

The gut–muscle axis is one of the more important emerging ideas in muscle ageing research, but its value lies in careful interpretation rather than exaggerated claims. Your gut does not replace the better-established drivers of muscle preservation, and it does not act as a hidden master switch that determines muscle fate on its own. What it appears to do is help shape the internal environment in which muscle is either maintained or gradually lost. That includes influencing inflammation, barrier integrity, microbial metabolite production, nutrient handling, and the broader metabolic setting in which muscle tissue responds to food, activity, and ageing.

This matters because muscle decline rarely develops through one isolated pathway. As discussed throughout this book, sarcopenia tends to emerge when multiple pressures begin to reinforce each other. Activity may fall. Appetite may narrow. diet quality may weaken. Chronic low-grade inflammation may rise. Recovery may become less efficient. The gut sits within that network rather than outside it. When the gut environment becomes less favourable, it may add to the biological load that makes muscle preservation harder over time.

One of the most useful lessons from this chapter is that gut health and muscle health should not be treated as unrelated topics. The same broad patterns that support one often support the other. A dietary pattern built around meaningful protein, fibre-rich plant foods, and mostly minimally processed staples is already moving in a direction that supports a healthier gut environment while also helping protect muscle. In that sense, the chapter does not point you toward a completely separate strategy. It deepens your understanding of why the basics matter.

At the same time, this chapter should leave you with discipline as well as interest. The evidence for gut-targeted interventions is promising, but not yet strong enough to justify hype. Probiotics, prebiotics, synbiotics, and related approaches may eventually play a more defined role in sarcopenia prevention or management, but they are not a substitute for the fundamentals. At present, they are best viewed as potential supports within a broader plan, not as the centre of it.

If there is one practical takeaway, it is this: muscle is easier to preserve in a body with a stronger internal environment. The gut may be one of the systems helping to shape that environment. Looking after it will not eliminate the need for training, protein, recovery, and a strong overall diet. But it may help create conditions in which those strategies work more effectively and more reliably across time.

The next chapter turns to the earlier adult years, exploring how muscle reserve is built and how it can be protected through the competing demands of midlife.

Chapter 10: Building Muscle Reserve in Early Adulthood and Protecting It in Midlife

Introduction

It is easy to think of muscle loss as a problem that belongs to old age. That is one reason so many people overlook the years when muscle reserve is actually being built, maintained, or quietly allowed to slip. By the time weakness, slower recovery, reduced physical confidence, or visible loss of muscle become obvious, part of the story has often been unfolding for years. Muscle ageing does not begin only when you feel old. It begins earlier, often quietly, and often without attracting much attention until the gap between what your body once did easily and what it now finds difficult becomes harder to ignore.

This matters because muscle is not only a tissue you notice when you are training hard, lifting something heavy, or trying to look leaner. It is reserve. It is capacity. It is what allows you to move well, stay independent, recover from setbacks, tolerate illness, maintain metabolic health, and meet the physical demands of ordinary life without feeling as though everything takes more effort than it should. The stronger that reserve is earlier in adulthood, the more protection you carry into later decades. The weaker it becomes through neglect, interruption, or slow lifestyle drift, the less margin you have when ageing, illness, injury, or inactivity begin to place more pressure on the system.

This is why midlife matters so much. It is not simply a stage that sits between youth and old age. It is often the period when competing demands begin to pull people away from the habits that once helped protect muscle. Training becomes less consistent. Sedentary time increases. Work and caregiving pressures accumulate. Sleep can worsen. Diet quality may drift. Weight may rise even while strength and muscle quality quietly decline. These changes do not always look dramatic from the outside, which is exactly why they are so often underestimated. A person may feel broadly functional and still be losing reserve in ways that only become obvious later.

That quiet drift is one of the most important ideas in this chapter. Muscle decline is not always the result of one major event. It is often the outcome of many smaller decisions, interruptions, and compromises that become normal over time. A few years of less training. More sitting. Less daily movement. More reliance on convenience. Repeated periods of stress and under-recovery. Weight gain without meaningful strength work. None of these factors guarantees poor outcomes on its own. But together they can gradually reshape the body into one that carries less reserve than it once did.

The encouraging part is that this process is not fixed. You do not have to be an athlete in early adulthood to build meaningful muscle reserve, and you do not need perfect habits in midlife to protect it. What matters more is direction. The body responds to repeated signals. If you train, move, eat, and recover in ways that support muscle, you can preserve far more capacity than many people realise. If those signals disappear for too long, the system adapts in the other direction. This makes muscle reserve both vulnerable and highly worth protecting.

This chapter focuses on that lifespan window. It explores what muscle reserve actually is, why early adulthood matters more than most people think, why midlife is often where protection becomes urgent, and how reserve is either preserved or eroded through the competing demands of real life. The goal is not to create fear about ageing. It is to make clear that the groundwork for later strength, resilience, and independence is laid much earlier than most people are led to believe.

What Muscle Reserve Actually Is

Muscle reserve is best understood as stored physical capacity. It is not just the amount of muscle you carry on your body at any given time. It is the margin between what your body currently needs to do and what it is capable of doing. That margin matters. It gives you room to cope with stress, illness, inactivity, recovery demands, unexpected setbacks, and the gradual physiological changes that come with age.

This idea is important because many people think about muscle in narrow terms. They think of it as appearance, body shape, gym culture, or athletic performance. But muscle reserve is more practical than that. It is what helps you tolerate time away from training without losing function too quickly. It is what helps you recover after illness or surgery. It is what gives you the strength to keep doing ordinary tasks when energy is lower, joints are stiffer, or life becomes more physically demanding. In this sense, muscle reserve is less about looking muscular and more about having enough capacity in the bank.

That bank is built most effectively when the body is younger and more responsive, but it is never entirely static. Reserve can be built, protected, eroded, or rebuilt to some extent across adult life. Early adulthood matters because it is a period when muscle mass, strength, and performance capacity are typically at their highest or still rising. That does not mean everyone reaches some perfect physical peak. It means the body is generally more responsive to training, recovery is often easier, and the opportunity to establish strong habits is greater. What you build during this stage does not guarantee lifelong protection, but it can make later decline slower, less severe, and easier to resist.

Reserve also needs to be understood in more than one dimension. Muscle mass matters, but it is not the only relevant measure. Strength matters. Power matters. Muscle quality matters. Physical function matters. A person can carry a reasonable amount of muscle and still have a shrinking reserve if strength, power, and movement capacity are declining. This is one reason muscle loss can go unnoticed for so long. People often assume that if body weight has not changed much, nothing important is happening. In reality, reserve may already be slipping through lower strength, poorer physical conditioning, rising fat mass, or reduced movement confidence.

This is especially relevant in midlife, because this is often when visible cues become misleading. A person may still feel young enough not to worry, yet their daily life may already be moving in a more sedentary direction. Formal exercise may become less frequent. Work may involve more sitting. Family and time pressure may squeeze out recovery and consistency. Body composition may begin to drift even without dramatic weight change. In that context, reserve can fall quietly, not because the body has suddenly failed, but because the signals needed to maintain capacity are no longer as strong or as regular as they once were.

Muscle reserve is also what makes ageing more or less forgiving. Two people can enter later life at the same age with very different reserves. One may have built and protected strength, lean mass, and movement capacity over decades. The other may have spent years in low activity, repeated disuse, weight gain, or inconsistent nutrition. Both are ageing, but they are not ageing from the same starting point. That difference matters because the person with greater reserve usually has more room to absorb the ordinary physical losses of ageing before they begin to affect independence and quality of life.

A useful way to think about reserve is as resilience made physical. It is the body's ability to withstand challenge without immediate loss of function. When reserve is strong, a setback does not cost as much. When reserve is weak, even a relatively short period of illness, inactivity, stress, or poor eating can have a much larger impact. This is why the chapter is not really about muscle in the aesthetic sense. It is about how much physical resilience you are carrying into the future.

Seen that way, muscle reserve becomes less abstract. It is not a concept only for researchers or athletes. It is directly tied to everyday life. It influences how easily you get out of a chair, climb stairs, carry weight, recover after time off, tolerate stress, and maintain independence as the decades pass. The more reserve you build and protect, the less vulnerable you are to the gradual narrowing of physical capacity that so often gets dismissed as "just ageing" when it is actually partly the result of years of underuse.

Why Early Adulthood Matters

Early adulthood matters because it is one of the most important periods for building the physical reserve that will support you later. This does not mean your body reaches a perfect peak and then simply begins to fall apart. The trajectory is more gradual than that. But these years are still critical because they are often when muscle mass, strength, movement confidence, and training responsiveness are at their strongest. In practical terms, this is when the body is most able to build capacity efficiently, and that capacity can act as protection in the decades that follow.

This is easy to overlook because early adulthood rarely feels urgent. Most people are not thinking about sarcopenia in their twenties or thirties. They are thinking about work, relationships, family, time pressure, body image, injury, or fitness goals that feel more immediate. Because the body is often still relatively forgiving at this stage, it is possible to assume that muscle takes care of itself. That assumption is one of the main reasons the importance of muscle reserve is missed. The consequences of underbuilding or underprotecting muscle are often delayed, which makes the issue feel less real than it actually is.

The value of early adulthood is not only that it allows you to build more muscle. It is that it helps establish a higher starting point. If you enter later decades with greater strength, more lean mass, better movement capacity, and stronger training habits, you are beginning from a more protected position. Age-related decline may still occur, but it takes longer to become functionally significant. In contrast, if early adulthood is marked by repeated inactivity, low strength, poor diet quality, or long stretches without meaningful loading, the body enters later life with less reserve in hand.

This is why muscle should not be thought of only as something to recover once it has already been lost. It is far easier to protect reserve than to rebuild it after years of decline. The body can regain capacity, but rebuilding usually becomes harder with age, not easier. This makes early adulthood less about chasing a cosmetic ideal and more about taking advantage of a window in which the body is highly responsive to training and adaptation.

There is also a behavioural reason these years matter. Early adulthood is often when long-term habits take shape. People establish whether resistance training is part of life or something done only in bursts. They develop patterns around food quality, protein intake, sleep, alcohol, stress, and movement. These habits may not seem dramatic in the short term, but over many years they help determine whether muscle is being steadily supported or gradually neglected. A person does not need to live perfectly for these habits to matter. What matters is whether the broad direction supports strength and physical capacity or quietly works against them.

Another reason early adulthood matters is that muscle decline does not always announce itself with obvious visual change. Strength and power can begin to slip before people recognise that anything meaningful is being lost. This means a person may assume they are maintaining well simply because they still feel generally capable. But capability in day-to-day life is not always the same as preserving reserve. It is possible to remain functional while still drifting downward from a stronger baseline.

This section is also important because it helps correct a common misconception: that muscle health only becomes relevant once you are older, injured, or visibly weaker. In reality, later-life strength is partly built on what was protected much earlier. The earlier adult years are not separate from the ageing story. They are part of it. They help determine how much buffer you carry into the stages of life when recovery becomes slower, interruptions become more costly, and the margin for error narrows.

In practical terms, early adulthood gives you a chance to make later life easier. Not effortless, but easier. The body you build and the habits you establish during these years can increase your resilience against inactivity, illness, stress, and the cumulative pressures of ageing. That is why these years matter so much. They are not only about present fitness. They are about future protection.

Midlife Is Where Protection Becomes Urgent

Midlife is often the stage when muscle preservation stops being a theoretical issue and becomes a practical one. Not because everyone suddenly becomes weak, but because this is often when the gap begins to widen between what the body could once handle easily and what it is now being asked to tolerate. Work becomes more sedentary. Recovery is less forgiving. Training consistency becomes harder to maintain. Sleep may worsen. Weight may drift upward. Stress becomes more chronic. None of these changes has to be dramatic to matter. Their effect comes from repetition.

This is what makes midlife so important. It is often the point at which muscle reserve begins to be tested more seriously, even if obvious decline has not yet set in. A person may still feel broadly capable and still be moving through life without major limitation, yet the conditions that protect muscle may already be weakening. Strength work may be less frequent. Daily movement may be lower. Meals may become more convenient and less structured. Recovery may be compromised by long workdays, caregiving demands, or fragmented sleep. Over time, these shifts can quietly reduce the body's margin of safety.

One of the reasons midlife is often underestimated is that the changes can be hard to see. Muscle decline does not always announce itself through sudden loss of independence or major physical failure. It often appears first as smaller changes that are easy to dismiss: feeling less spring in movement, slower recovery after training, reduced confidence with heavier tasks, more stiffness after inactivity, more difficulty returning to fitness after time off, or a growing sense that the body is less tolerant of inconsistency than it once was. These changes may sound minor, but they often signal that reserve is no longer being protected as well as before.

This is also the stage when body composition can become more misleading. A person may maintain a similar body weight for years and assume that little has changed, while underneath that stability muscle quality and strength may be worsening and fat mass may be slowly increasing. In other cases, body weight rises, but the added weight does not represent increased reserve. It reflects a body carrying more load with less functional protection underneath it. This is one reason midlife can become a turning point. The body may still look broadly familiar while becoming less physically resilient.

Midlife is also where interruption starts to matter more. In early adulthood, people can often bounce back quickly from periods of inactivity, poor sleep, or inconsistent eating. In midlife, that rebound tends to become less automatic. A few months away from training can cost more. Repeated stressful periods can have a greater effect. Illness, pain, work pressure, and family responsibilities can disrupt healthy habits for longer stretches, and the body may not recover from those disruptions as effortlessly as it once did. The same patterns that once seemed manageable begin to carry a higher physical cost.

For women, this period may bring an additional layer of vulnerability through the menopausal transition, when hormonal changes can affect muscle mass, strength, power, and body composition. That does not mean midlife in women should be framed as inevitable decline, but it does mean that protection becomes even more important. The broader point remains the same for both men and women: midlife is when many people first begin to feel the combined effect of reduced training consistency, changing recovery biology, lifestyle drift, and accumulating physiological stress.

This is why midlife should not be treated as a waiting room before older age. It is a decisive stage. It is the period when muscle reserve is either actively protected or gradually surrendered. The encouraging part is that this process is still highly responsive to change. Midlife is not too late. In many ways, it is exactly the right time to become deliberate. When people strengthen their training habits, improve daily movement, eat more consistently, recover better, and stop assuming their body will simply hold the line on its own, they often preserve far more capacity than they expect.

In practical terms, midlife is where prevention becomes urgent because the body is beginning to give clearer feedback. It is no longer enough to assume that being "not old yet" is protective. This is the stage when the quiet erosion of reserve can either continue unnoticed or be interrupted on purpose. The difference between those two paths can shape not only how you feel in midlife, but how much strength, resilience, and independence you carry into the decades that follow.

The Habits That Protect Reserve

Muscle reserve is not protected by one perfect habit. It is protected by the steady pattern of what you do often enough for your body to recognise it as normal. That is why this chapter matters so much. By midlife, many people are no longer losing capacity because they made one bad decision. They are losing it because life has slowly crowded out the habits that once helped them feel strong, capable, and physically at ease in their own body.

The most important of these habits is resistance training. As discussed earlier in this book, muscle is highly responsive to mechanical demand. If you give it a reason to stay, it is far more likely to remain. If you stop asking much of it, the body adapts in the other direction. This is one reason reserve can erode so quietly. You do not need to stop moving altogether to lose strength. You simply need to stop challenging it often enough. A busy life can create exactly that pattern: still active enough to get through the day, but not active in ways that meaningfully preserve muscle.

This matters because many people reach midlife with the impression that they are still "doing a fair bit," yet they are no longer doing the kind of movement that protects reserve. Walking is valuable. Staying generally active is valuable. But muscle also needs load, effort, and repetition. Without those signals, it becomes harder to maintain the strength and power that later protect independence, confidence, and resilience. This is why strength training remains so central. It is not just exercise for appearance or sport. It is one of the clearest ways of telling the body to keep its capacity.

Daily movement also matters more than many people realise. Formal training can help build and protect reserve, but long hours of sitting, low incidental movement, and repeated sedentary days can still work against it. The body responds to the full pattern of life, not only to isolated workouts. A person who trains a few times a week but spends the rest of life in prolonged inactivity is still sending mixed signals. In contrast, a person who stays physically engaged across the day often creates a more supportive environment for muscle, mobility, and metabolic health.

Food habits matter in the same way. Reserve is easier to protect when your meals consistently support the tissue you are asking your body to keep. That does not mean eating perfectly. It means not allowing years to pass in a pattern of poor protein intake, erratic meal structure, low diet quality, or repeated under-fuelling. As discussed earlier in this book, muscles do not only need exercise. They need adequate nutritional support to repair, adapt, and hold their ground. Midlife is often where this becomes more important because recovery is less forgiving and the body becomes less tolerant of long periods of nutritional neglect.

Recovery habits belong in this conversation too. Sleep, stress regulation, and the ability to recover from training and daily demands all influence whether reserve is being protected or slowly worn down. Many people in midlife are trying to carry heavy work, family, financial, and emotional loads all at once. That reality matters. A body under chronic stress and poor recovery is not functioning in the same environment as one that is consistently restored. This does not mean people need ideal conditions before they can protect muscle. It means that recovery is not optional background scenery. It is one of the conditions that helps good training and nutrition actually pay off.

There is also an emotional truth in all of this. The habits that protect reserve are often the very habits that make people feel more like themselves. Feeling strong enough to carry things without hesitation. Getting up from the floor without effort. Trusting your body to cope with a busy day. Not feeling fragile after a small setback. These are not trivial experiences. They shape confidence. They shape independence. They shape whether your body feels like something you can rely on or something you are slowly negotiating with.

This is why consistency matters more than intensity for most people. Reserve is not usually lost because someone failed to train like an athlete. It is lost because the basics stopped happening often enough. Strength work became occasional. Meals became rushed and less supportive. Sleep became chronically compromised. Days became more sedentary. The body adapted exactly as bodies do, to the life it was repeatedly given.

The encouraging part is that these same habits can begin to protect reserve again as soon as they become regular. You do not need to reclaim everything at once. You need to start sending clearer signals. Lift regularly. Move more across the day. Eat in a way that supports muscle. Recover as well as life realistically allows. Those actions may seem ordinary, but over time they are what separate a body that quietly narrows from one that keeps more of its strength, capacity, and freedom.

In practical terms, the habits that protect reserve are not glamorous. They are repeatable. And that is exactly why they matter. They keep you connected to your physical capacity long before loss becomes obvious, and they make it far more likely that the decades ahead will feel stronger, steadier, and less limited than they otherwise might.

Disuse, Body Composition Drift, and the Quiet Erosion of Capacity

For many people, muscle reserve is not lost in one obvious collapse. It is worn down more quietly. A few years of less training. Longer hours sitting. More fatigue at the end of the day. More interruptions, more time "just getting through the week," and less of the kind of movement that once kept the body feeling capable and responsive. This is one of the reasons muscle decline can be so hard to notice while it is happening. Life still functions. Work still gets done. Responsibilities are still met. But underneath that surface, capacity may already be narrowing.

Disuse is one of the most powerful drivers of this change. Muscle is expensive tissue for the body to maintain, and if it is not being used meaningfully, the body has little reason to keep investing in it. That does not mean you need to become completely inactive for losses to occur. More often, the shift is subtler than that. Daily life becomes less physically demanding. Incidental movement falls. Formal exercise becomes irregular. Strength work disappears first, then effort, then confidence. The body adapts to what it is repeatedly asked to do, and if the demand becomes too low for too long, reserve begins to erode.

What makes this particularly important in midlife is that the body often stops forgiving interruption as easily as it once did. In younger years, a few months off training may feel inconvenient but recoverable. In midlife, the same interruption can leave a more noticeable mark. Strength can fall faster than expected. Fitness feels harder to regain. Stiffness lingers longer. The return to previous capacity no longer happens automatically. This can be confronting, especially for people who still think of themselves as broadly fit or capable. The body may no longer be willing to absorb neglect without consequence.

Body composition drift adds another layer to the problem. Many people assume that if their body weight has not changed dramatically, they are holding steady. But body weight can stay relatively stable while muscle quality declines, fat mass increases, and physical capacity slips. In other cases, weight gradually rises, but that extra weight does not represent protection. It can instead mean the body is carrying more load with less useful reserve underneath it. This is one reason midlife can feel confusing. A person may still recognise themselves in the mirror while feeling increasingly unlike themselves in movement, energy, and resilience.

That quiet change can be emotionally unsettling, even when people do not talk about it in those terms. It may show up as a growing hesitation around tasks that once felt easy. A reluctance to lift heavier things. A sense that the body tires more quickly than it should. The frustration of feeling more out of shape than your age on paper seems to justify. These experiences matter because they are often early signs that reserve is being lost, not simply that life is busy.

Sarcopenic obesity is part of this same conversation. A person can gain fat mass while losing muscle quality and strength, creating the appearance of size without the protection of real physical capacity. That matters because excess body fat does not shield you from muscle decline. In many cases, it may compound the problem by increasing inflammatory burden, worsening metabolic health, and making movement feel harder. This is another reason body weight alone is such a poor guide to muscle reserve. It tells you very little about how much usable strength, power, and resilience you are actually carrying.

Disuse also tends to become self-reinforcing. The less strong you feel, the less likely you are to challenge the body. The less you challenge it, the more capacity slips. As capacity slips, everyday tasks feel more demanding, and the threshold for fatigue becomes lower. Over time, this can create a life that feels smaller physically without there ever having been one defining moment of decline. That is how reserve is often lost: not through drama, but through quiet narrowing.

This is why repeated interruptions matter so much. Illness, injury, work stress, long sedentary periods, pain, caregiving demands, and poor sleep do not simply affect the body while they are happening. They can leave a residue if they disrupt training and movement for long enough. One interruption may be manageable. But when interruptions become the norm and recovery periods are no longer followed by a strong return to meaningful physical demand, the body begins to settle into a lower-capacity state.

The important message here is not that every setback is dangerous. It is that disuse carries a cost, and that cost rises when it is repeated, prolonged, or normalised. The body can recover from interruption, but it does better when interruption is treated as temporary and followed by a deliberate return to movement, strength, and structure. When inactivity becomes the new baseline, the body adapts accordingly.

In practical terms, the quiet erosion of capacity often looks ordinary while it is happening. That is exactly why it deserves attention. The issue is not whether life gets busy. Of course it does. The issue is whether busyness slowly becomes a life in which strength, muscle, and movement are no longer being asked to stay. When that happens, the body listens.

Menopause and Muscle Vulnerability

For women, midlife can bring an added layer of complexity to muscle preservation. The menopausal transition is often discussed in terms of hot flushes, bone health, or reproductive hormones, but its effects do not stop there. It can also influence muscle mass, strength, power, recovery, body composition, and the broader sense of physical steadiness in the body. That does not mean menopause should be treated as a guarantee of rapid decline. But it does mean this stage deserves direct attention rather than being folded vaguely into "normal ageing."

One of the reasons this matters is that many women reach midlife already carrying the same pressures described earlier in this chapter: inconsistent training, long sedentary workdays, poor sleep, caregiving responsibilities, stress, and less time to recover well. When hormonal shifts are added to that background, muscle becomes more vulnerable not because the body suddenly fails, but because several pressures begin to stack on top of each other. Strength may become harder to maintain. Body composition may change more easily. Power and movement confidence may feel less automatic. Recovery may no longer feel as reliable as it once did.

This can be a confusing and frustrating experience. A woman may still be doing many of the same things she has always done and yet feel as though her body is responding differently. Muscle may seem harder to build. Fat gain may occur more easily, especially around the midsection. Strength may slip more quickly during time away from training. That shift is not imagined, and it is not simply a matter of willpower. It reflects a real physiological transition that can affect the musculoskeletal system as well as the hormonal one.

This is one reason menopause needs to be approached carefully in a book like this. It should not be framed as a catastrophe, and it should not be used to push simplistic promises. But it should also not be minimised. For some women, this stage becomes one of the clearest moments when muscle protection stops being optional and starts feeling necessary. The body is giving different feedback, and that feedback deserves to be heard.

The encouraging part is that muscle remains responsive. Resistance exercise continues to be one of the most effective tools for preserving and improving muscle mass and strength in postmenopausal women. That matters because it reinforces one of the central themes of this book: the body is adaptable, even when the biological environment is changing. Menopause may increase vulnerability, but it does not remove the capacity for improvement. In many cases, it makes regular strength-focused habits more important, not less effective.

This also helps correct a common misunderstanding. Some women interpret midlife physical changes as proof that nothing works anymore. In reality, the issue is often not that muscle has become untrainable. It is that the body now requires more deliberate support. The margin for autopilot narrows. Habits that once felt optional start to matter more. Strength training, adequate protein, movement across the day, and recovery become more protective because the background conditions are less forgiving.

Hormone therapy is sometimes discussed in this context, but the evidence does not support treating it as a simple answer for sarcopenia or muscle preservation. Its role is more nuanced than that, and the research is not consistent enough to justify strong claims that it should be viewed as a primary muscle strategy. This is important because women deserve a clear explanation rather than overselling. Hormonal change matters, but the practical foundations of muscle protection still remain the same: resistance training, adequate nutrition, regular movement, and attention to recovery.

There is also an emotional dimension here that should not be ignored. Midlife can be the point when some women begin to feel less at home in their own body, not because they have done something wrong, but because the body no longer feels as predictable as it once did. That loss of predictability can affect confidence as much as it affects strength. It can make women question whether decline is inevitable or whether it is even worth trying to resist. This is exactly where a more informed perspective becomes powerful. The body may be changing, but it is still highly worth investing in.

In practical terms, the goal is not to fight menopause as though it were an enemy. The goal is to recognise it as a stage where muscle vulnerability may increase and where deliberate protection becomes especially valuable. When women understand that this transition affects more than symptoms alone, they are in a stronger position to respond early rather than waiting until loss becomes harder to reverse.

Conclusion

Muscle reserve is one of the most important forms of physical protection you carry through life, yet it is rarely treated that way until it has already begun to shrink. This chapter has shown that the groundwork for later strength, resilience, and independence is laid much earlier than most people realise. Early adulthood is not only a stage of physical potential. It is a stage of accumulation. It is when reserve can be built more easily, habits can be established more deeply, and the body can be given a stronger starting point for the decades ahead.

Midlife then becomes the stage where that reserve is either protected or quietly allowed to erode. As discussed throughout this chapter, the change is often subtle at first. Strength work becomes less regular. Daily movement declines. Recovery becomes less forgiving. Body composition drifts. Interruptions last longer and cost more. For women, menopause may add another layer of vulnerability that makes muscle protection even more important. None of these shifts needs to be dramatic to matter. Their significance comes from how steadily they reshape the body over time.

That is why muscle reserve should not be thought of as a luxury or a fitness extra. It is part of how you stay capable in your own life. It affects not only how strong you are, but how well you tolerate stress, recover from setbacks, carry out ordinary tasks, and maintain confidence in your body as you age. The more reserve you build and protect, the more room you have when life becomes physically demanding, when recovery is slower, or when the unexpected happens.

The encouraging message is that this is not a chapter about inevitability. It is a chapter about direction. You do not need perfect habits in early adulthood to benefit later, and you do not need to wait for obvious decline before you act in midlife. Muscle responds to what you repeatedly ask of it. When you train with purpose, move regularly, eat in ways that support muscle, and recover as well as life realistically allows, you are not only improving the present. You are shaping the physical margin that will support you later.

If there is one practical takeaway, it is this: later-life strength is not built later in life alone. It is built much earlier, then either protected or neglected through the years when life gets busiest and the body is easiest to take for granted. The more deliberately you protect that reserve now, the more strength, freedom, and resilience you are likely to carry into the decades ahead.

The next chapter turns to older age directly, focusing on how training and nutrition can be used to protect independence when maintaining strength, function, and resilience becomes even more critical.

Chapter 11: Training and Nutrition for Older Age: Protecting Independence

Introduction

By older age, the goal of muscle preservation becomes more specific and more personal. Earlier in adulthood, much of the conversation is about building reserve and protecting it before decline becomes obvious. After 60, the focus shifts. Muscle still matters for all the same biological reasons discussed throughout this book, but now its value becomes even easier to recognise in everyday life. It shows up in whether you can move with confidence, recover after illness, catch yourself when you lose balance, get out of a chair without hesitation, carry groceries without strain, and remain physically independent in the face of normal ageing, not just ideal circumstances.

This is why training and nutrition in older age should not be framed as optional extras or as desperate attempts to "stay young." That way of thinking misses the point. The real issue is not youthfulness. It is capability. It is whether your body remains reliable enough to support the life you want to keep living. Strength still matters deeply, but it is no longer just about how much force you can produce in a controlled setting. It is also about how quickly you can respond, how steady you are when you move, how well you recover from interruption, and how much physical margin you still carry when something unexpected happens.

Older age also changes the practical reality of what muscle-preserving habits need to look like. Appetite may become less reliable. Recovery may take longer. Illness and interruptions may have a greater cost. Periods of reduced activity can erode capacity more quickly, and rebuilding after a setback may no longer happen automatically. That does not mean the body stops responding. It means the strategy has to become more deliberate, more realistic, and more durable under less-than-perfect conditions.

This is one of the most important ideas in the chapter. Training for older age should not depend on perfect weeks, perfect health, or perfect motivation. It should be built to survive the kinds of disruptions that become more common later in life. A useful program is not one that only works when everything goes right. It is one that still protects strength, balance, function, and confidence when life becomes messier. In the same way, nutrition should not be treated only as a matter of ideal targets on paper. It must also work in the context of lower appetite, reduced intake, illness, fatigue, and the practical realities of ageing.

There is an emotional side to this as well. For many people, older age is not frightening because of age itself. It becomes frightening when the body begins to feel less trustworthy. A missed step feels more consequential. A period of sickness costs more than expected. Confidence narrows. Tasks that once felt ordinary begin to require planning or caution. These are not small experiences. They change how a person moves through the world. They shape whether independence feels secure or increasingly fragile.

That is why this chapter matters. It is not about turning later life into a training project. It is about understanding how exercise and nutrition can help protect one of the things people value most: the ability to remain steady, capable, and self-reliant for as long as possible. The aim is not to chase youthful performance. The aim is to preserve function in a body that still deserves to be trusted.

This chapter explores that reality directly. It looks at why power and balance become more important in older age, why resistance training still works after 60, why minimum effective dose thinking becomes especially useful, why appetite and intake often become harder to manage, and how consistency can protect independence even when health events and recovery constraints make life less predictable. The message is not that later life has to be managed with fear. It is that it can be approached with more clarity, more strategy, and more physical confidence than many people have been led to believe.

Why Power and Balance Matter More Than Most People Think

When people think about ageing and exercise, they often think first about general strength. Strength remains important, but in older age power and balance become especially important because they are more closely tied to the movements that protect independence in real life. It is one thing to be able to produce force. It is another to produce it quickly enough to stop a stumble, regain your footing, rise from a chair smoothly, step over an obstacle, or react fast enough when something unexpected throws you off balance.

That speed of force production is what gives power its practical value. In younger adults, a modest decline in power may go largely unnoticed because reserve is still high and recovery is easier. In older adults, the loss becomes more meaningful because it affects exactly the kinds of fast, protective movements that keep people upright and confident. This is one reason power often matters more than people expect. It is not a specialised athletic concept. It is part of everyday safety.

Balance matters for similar reasons. Balance is not simply the ability to stand on one leg in an exercise class. It reflects how well the body coordinates posture, movement, strength, reaction time, and sensory input in real-world situations. When balance becomes less reliable, ordinary life can start to feel narrower. People may walk more cautiously, avoid uneven surfaces, become more hesitant with stairs, or lose confidence in settings that once felt routine. That loss of confidence matters because it can quietly reduce activity, and reduced activity then further weakens the very systems that support independence.

This is why falls should never be treated as random bad luck alone. Sometimes they are, of course. But often fall risk is shaped by the gradual interaction of weaker lower-limb strength, slower reaction time, poorer balance, reduced power, lower movement confidence, and less practice using the body dynamically. In that sense, falls are often not just accidents. They are warnings that reserve in the systems protecting movement may already be shrinking.

The encouraging part is that these qualities remain trainable. Evidence supports the value of exercise interventions that target strength, balance, and power in older adults, especially when the goal is preserving physical function and reducing fall risk. That matters because it shifts the discussion away from inevitability. If balance worsens and reactions slow, the answer is not simply to become more cautious and hope for the best. The answer is to train the capacities that help keep you steady.

This also changes how older adults should think about exercise. A walking program can be valuable, but it may not be enough on its own to protect the full range of abilities needed for independence. If an exercise routine does not ask the body to generate force, control posture, and respond dynamically, it may leave important gaps. That is why older-age training needs a broader purpose than "staying active." Staying active matters, but so does staying capable.

There is also a human reality here that many readers will recognise. What often unsettles people in older age is not simply feeling weaker. It is feeling less certain. Less sure of your footing. Less sure of how the body will respond if you trip, twist, move quickly, or land awkwardly. That uncertainty can change behaviour long before a serious fall occurs. It can make life smaller. It can turn ordinary movement into something more guarded and less free.

Power and balance training matter because they help resist that shrinking. They support the fast, steady, confident movement that keeps people participating in life rather than withdrawing from it. They do not guarantee that nothing bad will ever happen. But they do improve the physical conditions that make independence more likely and fragility less likely.

In practical terms, this means that exercise after 60 should not focus only on slow strength movements in predictable positions. Those still have value. But training should also help you move with control, react with more confidence, and maintain the kind of steadiness that protects you when life is not perfectly stable. That is why power and balance matter more than most people think. They are not extras. They are central to staying upright, capable, and independent.

Training That Still Works After 60

One of the most damaging ideas older adults absorb is that meaningful training is no longer realistic after a certain age. Some begin to believe they are too old to build strength. Others assume that if they cannot train the way they once did, there is little point in trying at all. Both views are deeply unhelpful. The evidence shows that resistance training still works after 60. Muscles remain responsive. Strength can still improve. Physical function can still improve. Balance can still improve. The issue is not whether training works. The issue is how it needs to be framed.

After 60, effective training often has a different purpose from the one it may have had earlier in life. The goal is usually not to chase personal records, dramatic physique change, or highly specialised performance. The goal is to maintain the physical qualities that keep everyday life manageable: getting up from a chair, climbing stairs, carrying weight, moving with confidence, recovering from setbacks, and reducing the risk that a health event turns into a lasting loss of independence. That shift in purpose is not a lowering of ambition. It is a sharpening of relevance.

This also means that older-age training needs to be judged by different standards. A useful program is not one that looks impressive on paper but cannot be sustained. It is one that produces meaningful strength and function while fitting the realities of the body and the realities of life. That may mean lower volume, more careful progression, more attention to joint tolerance, and a greater need for recovery between harder efforts. But none of that makes the training weak or unimportant. It makes it workable.

Combined approaches are often especially valuable here. Older adults do not usually benefit most from a program that isolates one physical quality while ignoring the others. Resistance training matters because it preserves and improves strength. Balance work matters because it improves steadiness and reduces fall risk. Power-oriented movements matter because they help maintain quick, protective reactions. When these are combined thoughtfully, training becomes more closely aligned with the actual demands of independent living.

This is one reason older adults should not assume that ordinary daily activity is enough on its own. Many people remain busy, but busyness is not the same as training. Daily activity may help maintain general movement, but it often does not provide enough load or challenge to preserve strength, power, and function at the level needed to resist age-related decline. The body adapts to what it is repeatedly asked to do. If it is never asked to work against meaningful resistance, it gradually becomes less able to meet demands when resistance appears unexpectedly.

There is also an emotional layer to this. For some people, the hardest part of training after 60 is not the body itself. It is the doubt that builds around the body. The fear of getting hurt. The feeling of being too far gone. The embarrassment of starting again. The quiet belief that strength belongs to younger people. These thoughts can make training feel like it is no longer "for you," even when it may be exactly what would help most. That is why the tone of this chapter matters. Older adults do not need to be spoken to as though their physical capacity is already finished. They need to be reminded that it is still worth asking something of the body.

This does not mean every older adult should train the same way. Health status, joint limitations, pain, mobility restrictions, confidence, and previous training history all matter. But the principle remains: training can still be effective even when it is adapted. A sit-to-stand can matter. A controlled step-up can matter. A loaded carry can matter. A resistance band movement can matter. A slower starting point does not make the work insignificant. What matters is that the body is being asked to stay capable.

Another important reality is that training after 60 often becomes more valuable precisely because the margin for error is smaller. When younger adults lose a little strength, daily life may barely notice. When older adults lose the same amount, the effect may be far more visible in balance, confidence, and function. That makes even modest improvements meaningful. A gain that looks small on paper may translate into far greater ease in real life.

In practical terms, training that works after 60 is training that can be repeated, progressed sensibly, and connected clearly to independence. It should challenge the body enough to preserve capacity, but not be so rigid or punishing that it disappears at the first sign of illness, fatigue, or interruption. Older age does not remove the value of training. In many ways, it reveals its value more clearly than ever. What changes is not whether it matters, but how directly its effects show up in the life you are trying to keep living.

The Minimum Effective Dose Mindset

One of the most useful ideas for older age is that training does not need to be maximal to be meaningful. In fact, one of the biggest reasons people lose momentum is that they imagine exercise only counts if it looks like a full, ideal program done under ideal conditions. That way of thinking can be especially damaging after 60, because life is less likely to offer uninterrupted months of perfect health, perfect energy, perfect motivation, and perfect routine. If training only "counts" when everything lines up, it becomes easy to stop altogether.

This is where the minimum effective dose mindset becomes so important. It shifts the question from "What is the perfect program?" to "What is the smallest amount I can do consistently enough to keep protecting my strength, function, and independence?" That is a far more practical question, and often a far more successful one. Older adults do not need training plans that collapse the moment travel, illness, poor sleep, joint flare-ups, or low-energy weeks appear. They need training habits that can survive real life.

This approach is not about lowering standards in a defeatist way. It is about protecting continuity. A shorter session still counts. One hard set still counts. A simpler routine still counts. A lighter training week during recovery still counts. These may not represent the highest possible training stimulus, but they can still be enough to preserve important physical qualities, especially when the alternative is doing nothing for weeks at a time. In older age, consistency often protects more independence than occasional bursts of ambition followed by long drop-offs.

This matters because interruption tends to cost more later in life. As discussed earlier in this book, the body usually rebounds less automatically with age. Time away from training can lead to more noticeable losses in strength, confidence, and function, and regaining that ground may take longer than expected. That is why the ability to keep some version of training alive through difficult periods is so valuable. It reduces how much ground is lost in the first place.

There is also an emotional relief in this mindset. Many older adults quietly carry the feeling that if they cannot do what they once did, then what remains is hardly worth doing. That belief can shrink effort before the body itself has truly given up. The minimum effective dose approach challenges that. It says that your body still benefits from being asked to do something meaningful, even if that "something" now looks smaller, simpler, or more carefully paced than it did years ago. That is not failure. That is intelligent adaptation.

This is especially important during illness, travel, pain flare-ups, caregiving periods, or emotionally difficult seasons. These are the moments when people often abandon structure entirely because they cannot manage their "normal" routine. But a body that loses all structure every time life becomes difficult is left more vulnerable each time. A body that keeps some signal going, even a reduced one, is more likely to hold onto capacity. This is where the minimum effective dose mindset becomes protective rather than merely convenient.

It also helps older adults avoid a common trap: overdoing it in a burst of motivation, then paying for it with extended soreness, fatigue, or discouragement. A smaller, sustainable amount of training often works better than an ambitious plan that exceeds recovery capacity. In older age, the best program is rarely the one that looks hardest. It is the one that can be repeated often enough to matter.

That does not mean progress becomes impossible. It means progress is often built from repeatable effort rather than dramatic effort. A manageable training week done regularly can preserve far more than a perfect month followed by two months of inactivity. A simple program you trust can be more powerful than a complicated one you cannot sustain. This is one reason the minimum effective dose mindset fits older age so well. It respects both the body's adaptability and the body's changing recovery realities.

In practical terms, this mindset asks you to stop treating disrupted weeks as lost weeks. If you are tired, train smaller. If you are recovering from illness, begin with less. If motivation is low, keep the session short but keep the habit alive. If a full program is unrealistic, protect the essentials. The goal is not to prove that you can train like a younger version of yourself. The goal is to keep enough stimulus in place that your body continues to recognise strength and function as necessary.

Over time, that way of thinking can make an enormous difference. It allows training to become something that bends without breaking. And in older age, a routine that bends without breaking is often what protects independence best.

Appetite Changes and the Nutrition Challenge of Older Age

One of the most misunderstood realities of older age is that nutrition often becomes more important at exactly the stage when eating well may become harder. Earlier in life, a missed meal, a low-appetite day, or a period of less structured eating may not seem especially significant. After 60, the margin for error often narrows. Appetite can become less reliable, meals may become smaller, illness may interrupt intake more easily, and the body may be less forgiving when protein and energy intake repeatedly fall short. This is one reason nutrition in older age needs more intention, not less.

The problem is not simply that older adults need nutrients. Everyone does. The problem is that the drive to eat may no longer match the body's needs very well. Hunger may feel weaker. Fullness may arrive sooner. Taste, routine, medication effects, dentition issues, fatigue, loneliness, grief, and illness can all change how food is experienced. For some people, eating begins to feel more like a task than a natural rhythm. When that happens, it becomes easy for intake to drift lower without anyone consciously deciding to eat less.

This matters because muscle is especially vulnerable when intake becomes unreliable. As discussed earlier in this book, muscle preservation depends on repeated nutritional support, particularly adequate protein. But older adults at risk of sarcopenia often consume less protein than those who maintain better muscle health. That does not always happen because they lack knowledge. Often it happens because appetite, energy, and routine no longer support eating in the way they once did. In that sense, the nutritional challenge of older age is often not theoretical. It is practical and deeply human.

There is also an emotional side to this that deserves to be acknowledged. Many older adults do not experience declining appetite as a dramatic health event. They experience it quietly. Meals become simpler. Portions get smaller. The motivation to cook fades. Eating alone becomes less appealing. Fatigue makes effort feel disproportionate. Over time, food can become less of a source of nourishment and more of something to "get through." That shift matters because it can gradually reduce not only intake, but the regular structure that helps protect muscle.

Protein becomes especially important in this context because the body still needs a strong nutritional signal even when appetite is weaker. This does not mean every meal must be large or mathematically perfect. It means older adults often benefit from being more deliberate about including meaningful protein in meals rather than assuming it will take care of itself. When appetite is low, this becomes even more important. A small meal with very little protein may fill the stomach without giving muscle much support. That is one reason meal quality often matters so much in older age.

This also helps explain why nutrition advice for older adults cannot rely only on ideal targets written on paper. A person may technically need more protein, but if appetite is low, chewing is difficult, cooking feels burdensome, or illness has disrupted routine, then the real question becomes how to make that intake feasible. This is where practicality matters. Sometimes protecting nutrition means using simpler meals, easier protein options, familiar staples, or repeated foods that are manageable and well tolerated. In older age, the best nutritional strategy is often the one that can still work on an ordinary, imperfect day.

Energy intake matters too. When overall intake falls too low, the body has less support for recovery, less protection during illness, and less flexibility when physical stress increases. This can be especially problematic during periods of unintentional weight loss, reduced mobility, or after hospitalisation. In these moments, a low intake is not just a temporary inconvenience. It can accelerate physical decline by making it harder to preserve both muscle and function. That is one reason nutrition in older age should not be framed only in terms of "eating clean" or avoiding excess. Sometimes the more urgent issue is simply eating enough, often enough, and with enough nutritional value to protect capacity.

There is also a common trap here. Some older adults continue trying to eat as though their main nutritional task is still weight control, even when the more important issue has become maintaining strength, recovery, and independence. This does not mean weight management suddenly stops mattering. It means the nutritional priorities may need to shift. If the body is getting smaller, weaker, less resilient, or less able to recover, then preserving nutritional adequacy becomes especially important. At that stage, under-eating can be far more harmful than many people realise.

This is why older-age nutrition often depends less on perfection and more on consistency. A few well-supported meals each day, each containing meaningful protein and enough overall nourishment, can do far more than occasional ideal eating mixed with long stretches of nutritionally thin intake. The body responds to what is repeated. If intake is repeatedly too low, too light, or too poor in protein, muscle pays the price over time.

In practical terms, older age often requires a more compassionate and deliberate approach to food. Not because older adults are fragile, but because their needs and realities change. Appetite may no longer be a reliable guide. Fullness may arrive too soon. Cooking may require more effort than before. Illness may disrupt eating more easily. Under those conditions, nutrition needs to be planned with more care, not left to chance. The goal is not to create pressure around food. It is to make sure the body still receives enough support to stay strong, steady, and capable for as long as possible.

Recovery Constraints and the Narrower Margin for Error

Older age does not make recovery impossible, but it does make it less automatic. This is one of the most important realities to understand if the goal is long-term independence. The body can still adapt, still improve, and still respond meaningfully to training and nutrition, but it often does so with a narrower margin for error. Sleep disruption costs more. Illness interrupts more. Time away from training leaves a deeper mark. Recovery after exertion may take longer. What once felt like a minor setback can begin to feel like something the body carries for longer than expected.

This matters because many older adults judge themselves against the way they used to recover rather than the way their body now actually functions. They expect to bounce back quickly, then become discouraged when soreness lingers, energy stays low, or strength does not return as easily after a break. That discouragement can become dangerous if it leads to the belief that the body is no longer worth investing in. In reality, the issue is often not that the body has stopped responding. It is that recovery now needs more respect.

As discussed earlier in this book, recovery is shaped by more than rest alone. Sleep quality, stress load, inflammation, illness burden, nutritional adequacy, and overall life strain all influence how well the body restores itself after effort. In older age, these pressures often begin to overlap more often. Sleep may be lighter or more fragmented. Medical issues may interrupt routine. Medications may affect energy or appetite. Illness may have a greater after-effect. Even emotionally difficult periods can reduce the body's ability to recover well. Under those conditions, a training plan that ignores recovery realities is unlikely to last.

This is one reason consistency becomes more important than intensity. A body with a narrower recovery margin usually does better with regular, manageable training than with occasional bursts of very hard effort followed by long periods of fatigue or inactivity. Older adults do not benefit from being repeatedly pushed into a hole that takes too long to climb out of. They benefit from a rhythm of effort that is enough to protect strength and function while still allowing the body to restore itself.

Illness is especially important here. In younger years, a short sickness may feel like an inconvenience. In older age, even brief illness can lead to noticeable declines in appetite, movement, strength, and confidence. That does not mean every illness causes lasting damage, but it does mean the cost of interruption can be higher. This is why the chapter has emphasised training and nutrition strategies that survive disruption. A body that has some structure to return to usually regains more ground than a body that slips into complete inactivity and under-eating every time health becomes unstable.

There is also a psychological burden in this stage of life that should not be ignored. Many older adults know what it feels like to lose a little ground and then realise how much effort it takes to recover it. That experience can create caution, and sometimes fear. A person may begin avoiding challenge not because they do not care, but because they know the recovery cost feels steeper than it used to. This makes thoughtful programming even more important. Training should feel demanding enough to matter, but not so punishing that it erodes confidence in the body.

Nutrition becomes part of recovery here as well. A body that is eating too little, especially too little protein, has far less support when illness, inflammation, poor sleep, or physical stress increase demand. This is one reason older adults cannot afford to think of food only as fuel for activity. Food is also support for repair. When recovery is less automatic, the body depends more heavily on regular nutritional help to hold onto muscle and function.

This narrower margin for error is also why small decisions begin to matter more. Going several days with poor food intake, long stretches of inactivity after a minor illness, or repeated nights of poor sleep may not feel dramatic in the moment. But in older age, those moments can accumulate more quickly into reduced strength, lower confidence, and slower movement. The body is still adaptable, but it no longer absorbs neglect as quietly as it once did.

In practical terms, this means older adults often need a more deliberate recovery mindset. That may include allowing more time between harder sessions, adjusting training volume when stress is high, restarting sooner but more gently after illness, protecting sleep where possible, and treating appetite loss as something important rather than incidental. None of this is about fragility. It is about realism. The more honestly recovery constraints are understood, the more effectively training and nutrition can be shaped around them.

Seen clearly, this is not discouraging. It is useful. It means that slower rebound does not have to be mistaken for failure. It means that setbacks do not need to become endings. And it means that older age can still be approached with a strategy that protects strength, steadiness, and independence, even when recovery no longer happens on autopilot.

Protecting Independence Through Consistency, Not Perfection

By older age, independence is rarely protected by one heroic effort. It is protected by what continues. It is protected by the habits that remain in place when motivation is low, when appetite is poor, when sleep has been disrupted, when the weather is unhelpful, when health has been unsettled, or when life simply feels heavier than usual. That is why consistency matters so much more than perfection. A perfect routine that disappears under pressure protects very little. A modest routine that survives real life can protect far more than most people realise.

This is an important shift in mindset because many people still judge themselves too harshly once life becomes less predictable. If they miss a week of training, eat poorly for several days, or lose structure during illness, they feel they have failed and may stop altogether. But older age does not reward all-or-nothing thinking. It rewards return. It rewards keeping enough structure alive that the body does not completely forget what it is being asked to remain capable of doing.

That principle applies to training first. A shorter session still helps. A simpler exercise day still helps. A return after interruption still helps, even if it begins below where you were before. Strength, power, and balance do not require theatrical effort to matter. They require repeated reminders. The body responds to those reminders over time. When they disappear for too long, independence becomes easier to lose. When they remain present, even imperfectly, the body is given a reason to stay capable.

The same is true of nutrition. A few days of lower intake do not define your future, but repeated periods of poor intake, very low protein, or appetite-driven under-eating can gradually weaken the body's support system. This is why consistency in older age does not mean dietary perfection. It means making sure the body is fed often enough and well enough that strength, recovery, and resilience have something to work with. A realistic nutrition pattern that continues through ordinary weeks is far more protective than a brief burst of ideal eating followed by long periods of nutritional drift.

Recovery belongs in this picture too. As discussed earlier in this chapter, older adults often live with a narrower recovery margin. That reality can feel discouraging if it is interpreted as loss alone. But it becomes more useful when it is seen as a reason to build steadier rhythms. The body does not need to be pushed to its limit every time to benefit. It needs enough support, enough movement, enough nourishment, and enough recovery to keep functioning well. In many cases, that quieter steadiness protects more independence than cycles of overexertion followed by shutdown.

There is also something deeply human in this section. For many older adults, what they want most is not a dramatic transformation. It is to keep doing ordinary things without fear or dependence. To keep walking confidently. To keep getting in and out of cars, beds, and chairs without hesitation. To keep carrying, climbing, reaching, gardening, shopping, travelling, and moving through daily life without that creeping sense that the body is becoming a problem to manage. These are not small ambitions. They are central to dignity and self-trust.

That is why consistency matters emotionally as well as physically. It helps preserve the feeling that your body is still yours to rely on. Each repeated walk, each strength session, each well-supported meal, each decision to restart after interruption reinforces the same message: this body is still worth maintaining. That message can be powerful, especially when ageing is too often described only in terms of decline.

Perfection, by contrast, can become its own kind of trap. It makes people wait for the ideal routine, the ideal motivation, the ideal week, or the ideal physical condition before they begin again. But older age does not always provide ideal conditions. Health fluctuates. Energy varies. Life interrupts. If the standard for success is perfection, many people end up doing far less than they are capable of. If the standard becomes consistency, even in simplified form, far more becomes possible.

This is why the habits discussed in this chapter should not be measured only by intensity or ambition. They should be measured by whether they help protect function. Does this way of training help you stay steady? Does this way of eating help you stay stronger through illness and recovery? Does this routine help you come back more easily after setbacks? Does it help you trust your body more rather than less? These are the questions that matter.

In practical terms, protecting independence through consistency means accepting that some weeks will be smaller than others, while refusing to let smaller weeks become permanent surrender. It means keeping enough structure in place that strength, balance, appetite support, and recovery remain part of life rather than occasional good intentions. Over time, that steady pattern becomes one of the most powerful forms of protection available in older age.

Conclusion

Older age changes the goal of muscle preservation, but it does not reduce its importance. If anything, it makes that importance clearer. By this stage of life, muscle is no longer just a matter of physical reserve in the abstract. It is part of whether you can keep living with steadiness, confidence, and independence. It affects how well you recover from interruptions, how safely you move through daily life, how resilient you remain after illness, and how much trust you still feel in your own body.

This chapter has shown that protecting independence after 60 depends on more than simply "staying active." Strength still matters, but power and balance become especially important because they influence the fast, practical, protective movements that keep people upright and capable. Resistance training still works, but it needs to be realistic enough to survive the realities of older age. Nutrition becomes more deliberate because appetite may no longer guide intake reliably. Recovery becomes more important because the body is often less forgiving of illness, poor sleep, under-eating, and long interruptions. All of these pieces matter because independence is not protected by one isolated strategy. It is protected by the way they work together.

One of the most important ideas in this chapter is that older age should not be approached with all-or-nothing thinking. Perfect routines are not what protect people most. Consistent routines do. A training habit that bends without breaking, a nutrition pattern that continues through ordinary weeks, and a recovery mindset that respects the body's changing needs can preserve far more function than many people expect. In later life, the body does not need perfection to benefit. It needs regular support.

This is also why the chapter has focused so strongly on daily life rather than performance for its own sake. For most older adults, the real question is not whether they can become exceptional. It is whether they can remain capable. Whether they can keep climbing stairs, getting off the floor, carrying what needs to be carried, staying steady when they move, and recovering enough from setbacks that life does not keep getting smaller. These are deeply practical goals, but they are also deeply personal ones. They shape dignity, self-trust, and quality of life.

The encouraging message is that later life does not remove the value of effort. It reveals it. A stronger body remains more protective. Better balance remains more protective. More reliable nutrition remains more protective. Better recovery remains more protective. Even modest improvements can matter when the goal is preserving independence, because in older age a little more strength, a little more steadiness, and a little more resilience can make everyday life meaningfully easier.

If there is one practical takeaway from this chapter, it is this: after 60, the aim is not to become younger again. The aim is to remain as capable as possible for as long as possible. That is not a small goal. It is one of the most worthwhile goals in the entire book. And it is still highly worth working toward.

Chapter 12: Injury, Pain, and Setbacks: Staying Strong When Training Isn't Perfect

Introduction

One of the hardest parts of protecting muscle across the lifespan is accepting that training rarely unfolds in a perfect straight line. Bodies hurt. Joints flare. Tendons complain. Illness interrupts momentum. Life becomes stressful. Motivation drops. Recovery does not always cooperate. For many people, these moments are where the real threat to long-term strength begins, not because the body has become incapable of adapting, but because setbacks so often trigger complete disengagement. A sore knee becomes no training at all. A pain flare becomes weeks of avoidance. A period of illness becomes a long drift away from movement. Over time, those stop-start cycles can cost more than the original problem itself.

This matters because muscle is not lost only through ageing in the abstract. It is often lost through interruption. The body adapts to what it is repeatedly asked to do, and when pain, fear, or discouragement lead to long periods of underuse, strength and function begin to narrow. That narrowing may feel justified in the moment. Rest seems sensible. Caution seems responsible. But when caution becomes deconditioning, the result is often a body that feels less trustworthy, less capable, and more vulnerable to the next setback.

That is why this chapter is so important. It is not about pretending pain does not matter, and it is not about pushing through everything recklessly. It is about learning how to keep some training signal alive when life and the body are no longer behaving ideally. It is about understanding that in many common conditions, especially arthritis and tendon problems, the answer is often not to stop moving completely, but to adjust the type, amount, or intensity of loading. It is also about recognising that setbacks are not only physical. They are psychological. They affect confidence, identity, and the belief that strength is still worth pursuing when the body no longer feels straightforward.

There is a quiet emotional weight to this that many readers will recognise. Few things are more discouraging than feeling as though every time you begin to rebuild momentum, something pulls you backwards again. A flare-up. A strain. A bad week. A painful joint. The sense that your body is becoming a negotiation rather than an ally. Over time, this can make people approach training with hesitation rather than trust. They begin waiting for the perfect pain-free window before they move again, and that window often never really arrives.

This chapter takes a different approach. It starts from the idea that successful ageing does not require perfect training conditions. It requires the ability to keep adapting when conditions are imperfect. That means understanding when pain does and does not mean stop, how to modify training through arthritis and tendon issues, how to reduce the damage caused by interruptions, and how to prevent setbacks from turning into a permanent loss of physical confidence. The goal is not to become fearless. The goal is to become steadier, more informed, and less likely to let temporary problems quietly become long-term decline.

When Pain Does and Does Not Mean Stop

Pain can be useful, but it can also be misleading. That is one of the reasons it creates so much confusion in training. People are often taught to think in extremes: either pain means damage and must be avoided at all costs, or pain is weakness and should simply be ignored. Neither view is especially helpful. Pain is real, important, and worth respecting, but it is not always a reliable sign that movement is harmful or that loading must stop completely.

This distinction matters because many common musculoskeletal problems do not behave like fresh trauma. A flare in arthritic pain, a sore tendon, or a long-standing shoulder or knee problem often involves sensitivity, irritation, and load intolerance rather than new structural harm each time discomfort appears. In these cases, the body may still respond well to training if the load is adjusted appropriately. That is why the more useful question is often not, "Does this hurt at all?" but, "What kind of pain is this, how much is it responding to load, and what happens if I modify rather than abandon the session?"

For many readers, this will already feel familiar. You start moving and something feels stiff or sore, but then it warms up and becomes more manageable. Or a joint feels worse after too much rest than after gentle movement. Or you notice that stopping completely for a week does not really solve the problem, but it does make you feel weaker, less mobile, and more hesitant. These experiences are important because they remind you that pain and harm are not always the same thing.

This does not mean pain should be dismissed. Some pain does mean stop or seek assessment, especially if it is sharp, escalating, associated with significant swelling, sudden loss of function, obvious instability, night pain that is new and severe, or symptoms that feel dramatically different from the usual pattern. But many flare-ups are less dramatic than that. They are often signs that the current load, volume, speed, range, or recovery state is not being tolerated well. In those cases, the answer is often to adjust, not disappear.

That idea can feel surprisingly emotional for people who have lived through repeated setbacks. Once pain has interrupted you enough times, it becomes easy to fear it. The body begins to feel unpredictable. A minor flare can feel like the beginning of another long decline. This is where a calmer framework becomes useful. Instead of treating all discomfort as danger, you begin to learn the difference between sensitivity and true warning. That change in interpretation can protect not only muscle, but confidence.

In practical terms, pain does not always mean a session has failed. It may mean you reduce the load, shorten the range, slow the tempo, choose a more stable variation, replace one movement with another, or shift focus for that day. A painful squat pattern might become a sit-to-stand. A heavy carry might become a lighter one. A tendon-irritating movement might be replaced with isometric work or a simpler alternative. These adaptations are not signs that training no longer counts. They are often exactly what keeps training possible.

There is also an important difference between pain during movement and pain after movement. Some discomfort during exercise may settle quickly and lead to no meaningful worsening afterward. In other cases, the session may trigger a flare that lingers too long or leaves function clearly worse. That response matters. It helps guide whether the current approach is tolerable or whether the body needs a smaller dose. This is one reason load management is so valuable. It turns pain from a reason to stop thinking into a reason to think more carefully.

The goal is not to make readers casual about pain. It is to stop pain from automatically becoming a doorway into deconditioning. When people interpret every flare as proof that they must stop, they often lose more from the long period of underuse than from the original problem. The body becomes less strong, less prepared, and more reactive. Then the next attempt to resume training feels harder, which reinforces the fear that movement is the problem. That is how stop-start cycles begin to accelerate decline.

A more useful mindset is this: pain may mean pause, modify, reduce, or reassess, but it does not always mean stop everything. Learning that distinction is one of the most important skills in long-term muscle preservation, especially for people living with recurring pain, stiffness, or flare-prone conditions. It makes training more realistic, more sustainable, and far less vulnerable to fear.

Arthritis and the Case for Adjusted Training

Arthritis is one of the most common reasons people begin to pull away from training, often long before they truly need to. A painful knee, a stiff hip, an irritable shoulder, or a flare after activity can make movement feel risky, and once that fear sets in, it becomes easy to assume that exercise is part of the problem. But in many cases, the opposite is closer to the truth. Well-adjusted exercise is often one of the most helpful things a person with arthritis can do for pain, strength, and function.

This is an important point because arthritis can feel emotionally discouraging in a way that goes beyond the joint itself. It can make people feel older than they are. It can make ordinary tasks feel uncertain. It can create the impression that the body is becoming brittle, when what is often happening is that the body has become more sensitive and less tolerant of poorly managed load. That distinction matters. A less tolerant joint does not always need total rest. Often it needs smarter loading.

This is where training needs to be reframed. The question is not whether someone with arthritis should train, but how they should train in a way the joint can tolerate and benefit from. Resistance training and other exercise interventions have been shown to improve pain, strength, and function in common forms of osteoarthritis, especially when the program is adjusted to the person rather than imposed rigidly. That matters because it helps replace the fear-based message of "protect the joint by doing less" with a more useful one: protect the joint by helping the body around it stay stronger and more capable.

For many readers, this will already match lived experience. A joint may feel stiffest after too much sitting. Pain may ease once movement begins. Confidence may improve when the leg or shoulder feels stronger. This does not mean arthritis is imaginary or that pain should be ignored. It means that complete avoidance is often not the answer. If the muscles surrounding a joint become weaker, movement becomes more guarded, and general activity falls, the body often becomes less resilient rather than more protected.

That is one reason strength matters so much in arthritis. Stronger muscles can help improve joint support, reduce the effort required for everyday tasks, and make movement feel more stable and less threatening. This is especially important in older age, where the cost of avoiding movement is often much greater. A person who stops training because of arthritis may not only lose tolerance in the affected joint. They may also lose balance, power, walking confidence, and independence more broadly. The body rarely deconditions in one isolated place.

This does not mean every exercise suits every arthritic joint. Load, range of motion, speed, exercise choice, and total volume all matter. A painful movement pattern may need to be shortened, slowed, supported, or replaced temporarily. A deep squat may become a sit-to-stand from a higher surface. A step-up may need a lower height. A painful pressing movement may need a different angle or lighter load. What matters is keeping some meaningful work going rather than allowing pain to eliminate all stimulus.

It is also worth acknowledging that arthritis pain is rarely influenced by mechanics alone. Fatigue, stress, poor sleep, inflammation, inactivity, and previous bad experiences with pain can all increase sensitivity. That is one reason a flare does not always mean damage has suddenly worsened. Sometimes it means the joint has been asked for too much, too fast, or under conditions the body was less prepared to handle. Responding well often means reducing and recalibrating, not surrendering.

There is emotional relief in understanding this. Many people with arthritis quietly fear that pain means their world must keep getting smaller. They begin avoiding hills, stairs, certain exercises, or even whole forms of activity because they assume the safest path is to do less. But doing less too often can become the very thing that makes the body less able to cope. A more hopeful and evidence-based message is that arthritis does not automatically end the training story. It changes the way the story is managed.

In practical terms, adjusted training usually means finding the highest level of tolerable loading rather than chasing either extreme. Too much can flare symptoms. Too little can leave the body weaker and less protected. The art is in working between those extremes. Some days that will mean a smaller session. Some days it will mean changing the exercise menu. Some days it will mean staying with simpler, more controlled movements. None of that is failure. It is how long-term training survives in a body that is not pain-free but is still highly worth strengthening.

Seen this way, arthritis is not a reason to abandon exercise. It is a reason to become more skilful with it. And in many cases, that skill can make the difference between a body that slowly withdraws from life and one that keeps enough strength and confidence to remain engaged in it.

Tendon Problems, Flare-Ups, and Smarter Loading

Tendon pain has a way of making people lose trust in movement. Unlike some injuries that feel dramatic and clearly defined, tendon problems often linger, fluctuate, and behave unpredictably. A movement feels manageable one day and irritating the next. Rest may calm things briefly, but too much rest often leaves the area feeling weaker, stiffer, and no more trustworthy than before. That is one reason tendon issues so often lead to stop-start cycles. People either push too hard and flare things up, or rest too completely and return with less tolerance than they had before.

This is where smarter loading becomes essential. In many tendon problems, the goal is not total rest unless symptoms are truly severe or something more acute is going on. The goal is to find a level of loading the tendon can tolerate and gradually adapt to. Tendons usually respond best when they are given a reason to improve without being repeatedly overwhelmed. That makes the strategy different from both extremes: it is neither push through recklessly nor shut everything down.

This distinction matters because tendon pain can feel emotionally exhausting. It is often one of the conditions that makes people feel trapped between fear and frustration. If they move, they worry they are making it worse. If they stop, they feel themselves getting weaker and less capable. Over time, this can create a kind of training hesitation where every session feels like a gamble. That hesitation is understandable, but it often becomes part of the problem if it leads to long-term underloading.

What tends to help more is a calmer and more structured approach. Instead of asking whether the tendon is completely pain-free, the better question is whether the load is sensible, tolerable, and recoverable. Can you perform the exercise without a sharp escalation in symptoms? Does the tendon settle reasonably afterward rather than becoming markedly worse for days? Can the exercise be repeated consistently enough to create an adaptive signal instead of a repeated flare cycle? These questions are usually more useful than treating all pain as proof that the session has failed.

This is one reason isometric or otherwise simplified loading can be helpful during more irritable phases. They can allow the tendon and surrounding muscles to keep working without forcing the area through the kind of movement or speed that currently feels too provocative. The exact form will vary depending on the tendon involved, but the broader principle is the same: keep some training signal alive. A reduced signal is often far more protective than no signal at all.

Tendon problems also remind us that load is not only about weight. It is also about volume, speed, range, frequency, and recovery. A movement may be fine if it is slower, smaller, lighter, or done less often. It may flare when several of those demands are pushed at once. That is why smarter loading is often more effective than simply becoming more cautious. Caution on its own can drift into avoidance. Smarter loading keeps the body engaged while respecting current tolerance.

There is also an important time element here. Tendons often do not respond instantly. They may need patience, repetition, and steady exposure before they begin to feel more reliable. This can be difficult for readers who are used to judging sessions purely by how they feel in the moment. Tendon rehabilitation often requires thinking a little longer term. The question is not only whether the area feels perfect today. It is whether the broader pattern is moving toward greater tolerance, greater strength, and greater confidence over time.

This matters because full rest can become deceptively expensive. A tendon that is never meaningfully loaded does not usually become more resilient just because it has been protected from discomfort. More often, the body around it becomes less prepared, less strong, and less tolerant of future demand. Then when activity returns, the tendon may feel just as irritable, but the person is now deconditioned as well. That is exactly the kind of stop-start pattern this chapter is trying to prevent.

In practical terms, tendon problems are often managed best by adjusting the training dose rather than abandoning training altogether. That may mean swapping exercises, reducing speed, shortening range, lowering frequency, using isometrics temporarily, or shifting emphasis to nearby areas while the painful structure settles. None of that means progress has stopped. It means the plan has become more intelligent.

Seen clearly, tendon flare-ups do not mean strength work is over. They mean the body is asking for better pacing, better load selection, and more patience. When that message is understood well, tendon pain becomes less of a dead end and more of a problem that can be worked around without letting the whole training habit collapse.

Avoiding the Stop-Start Trap

One of the most common ways people lose strength is not through one major injury, but through repetition of a familiar pattern: stop, rest, wait, feel weaker, try to restart, flare up, stop again. Over time, this cycle can become more damaging than the original problem. The body loses load tolerance, confidence drops, and each attempt to return feels harder than the last. What began as a temporary interruption slowly turns into a way of living in which training is always restarting but rarely continuing.

This matters because the body adapts not only to exercise, but also to the absence of it. When training is interrupted repeatedly, especially in midlife and older age, the effects can show up quickly in strength, function, movement confidence, and general physical capacity. A few weeks of doing less may not seem dramatic in the moment, but repeated often enough, those gaps begin to add up. The result is a body that feels less capable, not necessarily because it has suffered one severe setback, but because it has never been given enough uninterrupted time to hold onto what it built.

This is one reason stop-start cycles can feel so discouraging. They create the illusion that effort is pointless. You work to build momentum, then pain or life interrupts, and it seems as though everything unravels faster than it should. That experience can make people wary of trying again. They begin approaching exercise with guarded optimism, expecting the next setback before the current progress has even settled in. In that state, it becomes easy to confuse interrupted progress with proof that progress is no longer possible.

But the real problem is usually not that the body has stopped responding. It is that the rhythm of training has become too unstable to let adaptation accumulate. Strength is built through repetition. So is confidence. So is tolerance. When each new attempt is separated by long gaps of rest, fear, or inconsistency, the body never fully settles into a stronger baseline. It is constantly being asked to begin again.

This is why setbacks need to be managed with continuity in mind. A flare-up does not have to become a full shutdown. A painful week does not have to become a lost month. A period of illness does not have to erase all training structure. The more successfully you can reduce rather than abandon, the less ground you usually lose. That may mean changing exercises, lowering load, shortening sessions, focusing on unaffected areas, or temporarily shifting to a smaller and more controlled routine. These choices can feel modest, but they often prevent the much bigger cost of complete disengagement.

There is also a physical reason this matters. When training disappears completely, muscles detrain, coordination becomes less sharp, joints can feel less supported, and general movement begins to feel less familiar. Then when the person tries to come back, the body is not returning from the same place it left. It is returning from a lower level of readiness. That lower readiness makes the next flare or overload more likely, which then reinforces the idea that training itself is the problem. This is how stop-start patterns become self-perpetuating.

The emotional side is just as important. Repeated interruption can slowly teach people to distrust their own body. They stop believing in momentum. They stop expecting consistency to be possible. They become more reactive and less deliberate, responding to every symptom spike as though it carries the same meaning. Over time, the issue is no longer just pain or injury. It is a shrinking sense of what the body can handle. Once that happens, life can begin to feel physically smaller even before major disability appears.

This is why the goal should never be to eliminate all interruption. That is unrealistic. Everyone gets setbacks. Everyone has painful weeks, stressful periods, illness, fatigue, travel, poor sleep, and life phases where training becomes harder. The real goal is to stop those interruptions from turning into a permanent rhythm of decline. A body can handle setbacks far better than it can handle surrender disguised as caution.

In practical terms, avoiding the stop-start trap means building a mindset that asks, "What can still continue?" rather than, "Does everything now need to stop?" It means recognising that a reduced version of training is often more protective than no training at all. It means returning sooner, even if more gently. It means understanding that consistency is not broken by adaptation. It is broken by disappearance.

Seen clearly, this is one of the most important skills in long-term muscle preservation. Not perfect training, but uninterrupted intention. Not never being set back, but knowing how to keep moving when setbacks arrive. That is what stops temporary problems from becoming a long-term physical identity.

Keeping a Training Signal Alive During Setbacks

The body does not need a perfect training week to hold onto capacity. It needs a reason to keep doing so. That is what a training signal is: a repeated reminder that strength, movement, and function are still needed. During setbacks, that signal may need to become smaller, simpler, or more carefully paced, but it is often far better to keep some version of it alive than to let it disappear completely.

This matters because many people still think in terms of all or nothing. If they cannot complete their full routine, they assume the session is no longer worth doing. If one area is painful, they stop loading everything. If life becomes chaotic, they wait for a future week when conditions will be better. But setbacks rarely work that neatly. The ideal week often does not arrive when hoped for, and in the meantime the body is adapting to less challenge, less coordination, and less confidence. A smaller signal maintained through a difficult period can protect far more than a total break followed by an uncertain restart.

Keeping a training signal alive does not mean pretending the setback is not real. It means responding in a way that protects continuity. A painful lower-body movement pattern may mean focusing more on upper-body work, trunk control, or simpler leg exercises for a time. A tendon flare may mean reducing range, speed, or volume while keeping some load in place. Arthritis may mean shorter sessions, more controlled movements, or lower impact options rather than no movement at all. Illness recovery may mean beginning again with very small doses instead of waiting until the body feels completely normal. These are not compromised versions of training in a negative sense. They are the version that keeps the habit alive.

This is where minimum effective dose thinking becomes especially useful. During setbacks, the goal is often not to progress aggressively. The goal is to avoid falling all the way back to zero. One or two meaningful exercises may be enough for that period. One hard set may be enough for that period. A shorter walk, a chair-based movement session, some controlled sit-to-stands, a few loaded carries, or a brief band routine may be enough for that period. These efforts can look unimpressive from the outside, but their effect over time can be surprisingly important because they maintain contact with strength, movement, and effort.

There is also an emotional benefit to this. When people keep some signal alive, they are less likely to feel as though they have "lost everything" every time life goes off track. The setback becomes something they are working through rather than something that has taken the whole training habit away. That distinction matters. It protects identity as much as physiology. A person who continues doing something usually feels closer to return than a person who has stopped entirely and now has to overcome both physical detraining and the psychological weight of starting over again.

This is particularly important for older adults, but it applies across the lifespan. The narrower the recovery margin, the more valuable continuity becomes. If a person loses several weeks every time a flare-up happens, those lost weeks accumulate quickly. If instead they learn how to scale training while staying engaged, the body retains more readiness and the next step back toward fuller training becomes easier.

A training signal can also be maintained through focus shifts. If one region is irritated, another may still be trainable. If heavy loading is not tolerated, slower tempo or supported movement may still work. If fatigue is high, the session may become shorter rather than disappearing. This is one reason a flexible approach is so important. The question during setbacks is not whether the original plan can be executed perfectly. The question is what still gives the body a useful reason to stay strong.

In practical terms, keeping a training signal alive often means protecting a few essentials. Maintain some resistance. Maintain some movement. Maintain some routine. Maintain some intention. The body responds to those cues even when they are reduced. When they vanish entirely, detraining begins to do its work quietly and quickly.

That is why setbacks should not only be measured by how much pain or inconvenience they bring. They should also be measured by how much structure they remove. If structure can be preserved, even in a smaller form, muscle and confidence are both more likely to survive the interruption. Over time, that may be one of the most powerful differences between people who keep ageing with strength and those who gradually drift into lower-capacity living without ever meaning to.

The Psychology of Setbacks

Pain and interruption do not affect only the body. They change the way people think about the body. That change can be just as important as the physical setback itself. A painful flare, a failed return to training, or a setback that lasts longer than expected can quietly teach a person to become more cautious, more doubtful, and less willing to trust movement. Over time, the issue is no longer only whether the knee hurts or the tendon is irritated. The issue becomes whether the body still feels like something safe to rely on.

This is one of the reasons setbacks can have such a lasting effect. They often reshape confidence before they reshape capacity completely. A person may begin avoiding certain movements, then certain exercises, then whole categories of activity. They tell themselves they are being sensible, and sometimes they are. But sometimes what is happening is overprotection. The body is not being protected from harm so much as withdrawn from challenge. That withdrawal can feel safe in the short term, but over time it often leaves the person weaker, more hesitant, and less confident than before.

Fear plays a major role here. Once pain has disrupted you enough times, it becomes easy to expect the worst. You start scanning for trouble. A small ache feels like the start of another long setback. A stiff joint feels like proof that progress is collapsing. A missed session feels like the beginning of another failed attempt. This kind of thinking is deeply understandable, especially for people who have already lost ground more than once. But if it goes unchallenged, it can make the body feel permanently fragile even when it is still highly capable of adapting.

Discouragement matters too. Few things are more draining than feeling as though every time you build momentum, something knocks you back. That kind of repetition can make effort feel emotionally expensive. It can create the temptation to stop trying altogether, not because the person is lazy, but because they are tired of hoping and being disappointed. This is where many people begin telling themselves a story that is more damaging than the original pain: that their body is no longer worth investing in.

That story is rarely true, but it can become powerful if it is repeated often enough. It narrows possibility. It turns temporary symptoms into a permanent identity. A person stops seeing themselves as someone working through a setback and starts seeing themselves as someone whose body always goes wrong. Once that happens, training becomes harder not only because of the physical issue, but because of the meaning attached to it.

This is why rebuilding trust in the body matters so much. Trust is not restored by pretending pain does not exist. It is restored by repeated experiences of tolerable success. A session that is modified but completed. A movement that feels more manageable than expected. A flare that settles instead of spiralling. A week of consistency after a difficult month. These moments may seem small, but they matter because they teach the nervous system and the mind that movement is still possible, and that pain does not always have to end the story.

This is also why the tone of recovery matters. People often respond to setbacks by either becoming overly fearful or overly aggressive. One reaction is to avoid too much. The other is to try to regain everything immediately. Both can backfire. Rebuilding confidence usually works better when the body is given enough challenge to feel purposeful, but not so much that it feels repeatedly punished. A calmer progression often does more for long-term trust than a dramatic comeback attempt.

There is a human dignity in this process that should not be overlooked. When people lose trust in their body, they often lose more than fitness. They lose spontaneity. They lose ease. They lose the feeling that movement belongs to them rather than being something they must constantly negotiate. That is why rebuilding confidence matters. It is not only about returning to exercise. It is about returning to a more secure relationship with your own physical self.

In practical terms, the psychology of setbacks improves when the person stops asking, "Can I go back to exactly how I was before?" and starts asking, "What can I do now that moves me forward safely?" That shift changes everything. It moves the focus from loss to capability, from fear to strategy, and from all-or-nothing thinking to realistic progress. The body responds better when it is given this kind of steady, confident leadership.

Setbacks are real. So are frustration, fear, and disappointment. But none of those experiences has to become a final conclusion about what your body can still do. In many cases, the most important part of staying strong is not avoiding every setback. It is learning how to keep your confidence from collapsing when setbacks arrive.

Conclusion

Injury, pain, and interruption are not unusual detours from the muscle-preservation story. They are part of it. The question is not whether setbacks will happen. For most people, they will. The more important question is what those setbacks are allowed to become. They can remain temporary challenges that are worked around intelligently, or they can quietly turn into long stop-start cycles that erode strength, confidence, and function far more than the original problem ever needed to.

This chapter has shown that many common obstacles to training do not require total withdrawal. Arthritis often responds well to adjusted exercise. Tendon problems usually need better load management rather than full rest. Pain does not always mean damage, and it does not always mean that movement should stop. At the same time, setbacks do need respect. They ask for more skill, more patience, and more thoughtful progression, not denial. That is why the central message of this chapter is adaptation, not avoidance and not recklessness.

One of the most important ideas here is that repeated interruption carries a cost. When every painful flare, stressful period, illness, or difficult week leads to complete disengagement, the body begins to lose not only muscle, but readiness. Strength fades. Tolerance drops. Confidence narrows. Then the next return becomes harder, which makes the next setback more likely to trigger another withdrawal. This is how temporary problems become long-term decline. The physical losses are real, but so is the psychological shift that teaches a person to distrust movement and expect failure from the body.

That is why keeping a training signal alive matters so much. A reduced version of training is still training. A modified routine is still a routine. A smaller signal during a difficult period is often enough to preserve far more than people realise, especially when the alternative is weeks or months of doing nothing. This principle matters across the lifespan, but it becomes especially valuable in midlife and older age, when the body tends to lose more from disuse and recover less automatically than before.

There is also a deeper practical message running through this chapter. Staying strong when training is imperfect is not a lesser version of successful ageing. It is one of its central skills. Very few people move through life with uninterrupted momentum, pain-free joints, ideal recovery, and perfect consistency. Real success comes from learning how to keep going, even if in a different form, when life and the body are not behaving ideally. That skill protects muscle, but it also protects something equally important: trust in your own physical future.

If there is one practical takeaway, it is this: do not let every setback rewrite the whole story. Modify when you need to. Reduce when you need to. Rebuild more patiently when you need to. But keep some version of the signal alive whenever possible. A body that is imperfect can still become stronger. A body that hurts sometimes can still adapt. And a training life that is interrupted does not have to become a training life that disappears.

Chapter 13: Clinical Conditions That Accelerate Muscle Loss

Introduction

Muscle loss does not happen in a vacuum. It is shaped not only by ageing, but by the health conditions that change how the body handles energy, inflammation, movement, recovery, appetite, and adaptation. This matters because many people do not lose muscle simply because they are getting older. They lose it faster because chronic disease changes the internal environment in which muscle is trying to survive.

That shift is one of the most important ideas in this chapter. When conditions such as insulin resistance, type 2 diabetes, obesity, cardiovascular disease, osteoporosis, or chronic inflammatory disorders are present, muscle is often placed under pressures that go beyond ordinary ageing. The body may become less efficient at using nutrients, less responsive to anabolic signals, more inflamed, less active, more fatigued, or less able to recover from setbacks. Over time, those pressures can make muscle harder to maintain even when a person is trying to do the right thing.

This is why muscle should not be treated as a passive victim of chronic disease. It is often one of the tissues most affected by it. Muscle helps regulate glucose, supports movement, protects bone, contributes to metabolic health, and provides the physical reserve needed to cope with illness and stress. When muscle declines, chronic disease often becomes harder to manage. And when chronic disease worsens, muscle often declines further.

That two-way relationship is one reason muscle preservation becomes so important once health becomes more complicated.

There is also a practical and emotional reality to this. Many people living with chronic disease already feel as though their body is asking more of them than it used to. Energy may be lower. Movement may feel heavier. Recovery may take longer. Weight may change in frustrating ways. Confidence can shrink, especially when the body no longer behaves predictably. Under those conditions, it becomes easy to think of strength loss as inevitable or secondary. But in many cases, preserving muscle is not secondary at all. It is one of the most protective things a person can do.

This chapter is therefore not about giving a medical textbook description of disease. Its purpose is narrower and more useful. It asks a simpler question: how do these conditions accelerate muscle loss, and what does that mean for protecting strength, function, and independence? That is the lens through which each topic needs to be understood. Not as diagnosis for its own sake, but as muscle relevance.

This also means the chapter should be read with a practical mindset. The presence of chronic disease does not mean the muscle-preservation story is over. It means the strategy has to become more deliberate. Exercise may need to be adapted. Nutrition may need to be more intentional. Recovery may need more respect. Medication effects may need to be considered. And the body may need a little more patience without being let off the hook completely. In many cases, the goal is not to wait until health becomes ideal before acting. It is to protect as much muscle as possible within the reality of the health picture that already exists.

There is a deeper message here too. Chronic disease can make people feel as though their body is slipping away from them in pieces, one system at a time. But muscle sits at the centre of many of those systems. It is part of metabolic control, movement, resilience, and survival during illness. That is why it deserves direct attention. Preserving muscle in the presence of chronic disease is not cosmetic, and it is not optional background work. It is part of keeping the body more capable under more difficult conditions.

This chapter begins with one of the clearest examples of that relationship: insulin resistance and type 2 diabetes, where muscle is not only affected by disease, but deeply involved in it.

Insulin Resistance, Type 2 Diabetes, and Muscle Vulnerability

Muscle plays a central role in glucose control. It is one of the main tissues responsible for taking up and using glucose, especially after meals. That means muscle is not only affected by insulin resistance and type 2 diabetes. It is deeply involved in them. When muscle health declines, the body has less effective tissue available to help regulate blood sugar. And when insulin resistance worsens, muscle becomes harder to maintain. This creates a two-way relationship that can quietly accelerate decline in both directions.

This matters because many people still think of type 2 diabetes mainly in terms of blood glucose numbers, medication, or body weight. Those things matter, but they do not tell the whole story. Type 2 diabetes also changes the internal environment in which muscle is trying to survive. Impaired insulin action, chronic low-grade inflammation, altered nutrient handling, and reduced metabolic flexibility can all make muscle less responsive to the signals that normally support maintenance and repair. Over time, this can contribute to lower muscle mass, poorer muscle quality, and reduced strength.

That shift is important because muscle is not only a passive casualty of poor metabolic health. It is one of the main defences against it. A stronger, more active muscle mass helps improve glucose disposal, insulin sensitivity, and overall metabolic function. When that muscle reserve shrinks, the body loses some of its capacity to manage blood sugar efficiently. This is one reason the relationship between diabetes and muscle decline is so clinically significant. The problem does not move in one direction only. Each side can intensify the other.

There is also a practical reason this needs to be explained clearly. Many adults with insulin resistance or type 2 diabetes live with a gradual sense that their body no longer responds the way it used to. Energy may feel less steady. Fatigue may rise more easily. Physical activity may feel harder to recover from. Weight changes may become more frustrating. Strength may decline quietly. These experiences are not always discussed as muscle problems, but muscle is often part of the story. A body that is less metabolically efficient is often also a body that finds it harder to hold onto physical capacity.

Inflammation adds another layer. Type 2 diabetes is often accompanied by a chronic inflammatory burden that can interfere with muscle maintenance and adaptation. As discussed earlier in this book, muscle is easier to preserve in a body that is metabolically stable, nutritionally supported, and not under constant low-grade inflammatory stress. Diabetes can move the body away from that environment. This does not make muscle loss inevitable, but it does make muscle preservation more deliberate and more important.

There is a human side to this as well. People with type 2 diabetes are often told to focus on numbers, restriction, and disease management. What can get lost in that conversation is the experience of living in a body that may feel less capable than before. A person may notice they tire sooner, recover more slowly, or feel less physically confident, yet not realise that preserving muscle is one of the best ways to support both function and metabolic health. That misunderstanding matters because muscle can receive too little attention at exactly the time it should be protected most actively.

This is why exercise and nutrition remain so central. Resistance training, daily movement, and sufficient protein are not side issues for people with insulin resistance or type 2 diabetes. They are part of the strategy. A person does not need perfect metabolic health before building or protecting muscle. In many cases, muscle protection is one of the best supports available for improving the health picture overall. That does not make it easy, but it does make it worthwhile.

In practical terms, this section should leave the reader with one clear understanding: type 2 diabetes does not only affect muscle because disease is present. It affects muscle because it changes the conditions that muscle depends on. And once muscle begins to decline, the metabolic picture often becomes harder to manage. That is why the relationship deserves to be taken seriously. Protecting muscle in the presence of insulin resistance is not just about staying strong. It is part of helping the whole system function better.

Obesity, Sarcopenic Obesity, and Hidden Functional Decline

Obesity is often misunderstood in conversations about muscle. Many people assume that if body size is larger, muscle is automatically better protected. But that is not necessarily true. A person can carry more total body weight while still losing muscle quality, physical reserve, and functional strength. This is one of the reasons obesity can sometimes hide muscle decline rather than prevent it.

The term sarcopenic obesity is useful here because it describes a situation in which excess body fat coexists with lower muscle quality, lower strength, or lower functional capacity. This matters because the problem is not size alone. The problem is whether the body has enough usable, resilient muscle to carry that size well. A larger body without strong underlying physical reserve is not necessarily better protected. In some cases, it may be more vulnerable.

This is why body weight on its own can be such a misleading guide. A person may look substantial, may not appear "frail," and may even assume they are carrying enough mass to be safe from muscle loss. Yet underneath that appearance, movement may be getting harder, balance may be less secure, recovery may be slower, and strength may be declining in ways that are not obvious from the scale. That hidden functional decline is one of the most important things this section needs to bring into focus.

There is also a mechanical side to this. Carrying more body weight increases the physical demand of everyday movement, but that does not guarantee the body has the strength or power to manage those demands well. In fact, if muscle quality is worsening at the same time fat mass is increasing, daily tasks can become more tiring and less efficient. Stairs feel heavier. Walking becomes more effortful. Getting up from lower seats may require more strategy. The body is carrying more load, but not necessarily more useful reserve.

Inflammation and metabolic dysfunction add another layer. Obesity is often associated with a more inflammatory internal environment, and as discussed earlier in this book, chronic low-grade inflammation is not friendly to muscle preservation. It can interfere with anabolic signalling, worsen metabolic health, and make the body less responsive to the very inputs that would otherwise help protect muscle. This is one reason obesity and muscle decline can reinforce each other rather than cancel each other out.

This section is also important because the emotional experience of hidden decline can be confusing. A person may know they are heavier, but not fully understand why they feel less capable than before. They may focus only on body fat and miss the fact that muscle quality and reserve are also changing. Or they may attempt weight loss in ways that reduce overall body mass without protecting muscle well enough, leaving the body smaller but not necessarily stronger or more functional. That is why this chapter has to keep returning to the same core question: not just how much weight is present, but how much useful strength and function are present underneath it.

There is a strong practical implication here. In people living with obesity, muscle preservation should not be treated as secondary to body weight concerns. It should be part of the strategy from the beginning. Resistance training, adequate protein, daily movement, and recovery support become especially important because the aim is not merely to change size. The aim is to improve body composition quality, physical function, and metabolic resilience. A person does not become better protected simply by becoming lighter if muscle has been neglected in the process.

This is where a non-judgmental understanding matters. Obesity should not be discussed as personal failure, and sarcopenic obesity should not be framed in a way that shames the reader. The point is not to moralise body size. The point is to explain that muscle decline can be present in bodies of many sizes, and that larger bodies are not exempt from the need to preserve strength, power, and functional reserve. In fact, that preservation may be even more important when the body is already carrying greater mechanical and metabolic strain.

In practical terms, the most useful takeaway is this: obesity can conceal muscle vulnerability rather than protect against it. That is why the real focus should not be body weight alone, but whether the body remains strong enough, capable enough, and well-supported enough to function with confidence over time. When that perspective is understood, muscle preservation becomes part of the answer, not an afterthought.

Osteoporosis, Frailty, and Muscle–Bone Health

Muscle and bone are often spoken about as though they belong to separate conversations. Bone is treated as the issue of fracture risk, while muscle is treated as the issue of strength or sarcopenia. In reality, they are closely linked. They age together, fail together, and protect one another more than many people realise. This is why osteoporosis belongs in a book about muscle preservation. It is not a separate problem happening elsewhere in the body. It is part of the same story of physical resilience.

At the most basic level, bone depends on load. Muscle helps provide that load. Stronger muscles pull on bone, support movement, and contribute to the kinds of repeated mechanical signals that help maintain skeletal strength. When muscle declines, those signals often decline as well. The body becomes less physically demanding, less dynamically loaded, and often less stable. Over time, that makes bone loss and muscle loss more likely to travel together rather than separately.

This relationship becomes especially important in older age because the consequences overlap so closely. A person with weaker muscles is often less steady. A person who is less steady is often more likely to fall. A person with more fragile bones is less protected when a fall occurs. In that sense, osteoporosis is not only a bone-density issue. It becomes a muscle issue, a balance issue, and an independence issue. The risk is not just that the skeleton is weaker. The risk is that the whole physical system becomes less able to tolerate ordinary life without serious consequence.

That is one reason frailty often sits near the centre of this discussion. Frailty is not simply a matter of age. It reflects shrinking reserve across multiple systems, and the muscle–bone relationship is one of the clearest examples of that. When strength declines, confidence often declines with it. Activity becomes more cautious. Load-bearing movement may reduce. Fear of falling may lead to further inactivity. Bone and muscle then receive even less stimulus, and the cycle continues. This is how people can move from mild vulnerability to much more obvious decline without one single dramatic turning point.

There is also a practical misunderstanding here that needs correcting. Many people think of osteoporosis mainly as something to monitor medically rather than something connected to everyday function. But the real-life effect of osteoporosis is shaped heavily by what the muscles around the skeleton are still able to do. Stronger legs, better balance, faster reactions, and more controlled movement may reduce falls and improve the body's ability to manage daily demands more safely. That does not make muscle a substitute for bone health care, but it does make muscle preservation one of the most relevant parts of the picture.

This can feel emotional for readers because osteoporosis often changes how safe the world feels. A missed step, a slippery floor, a sudden loss of balance, or even the thought of falling can start to carry more psychological weight. People may begin to move more cautiously, do less, or avoid certain activities altogether. That response is understandable, but if it leads to chronic underloading, the body usually becomes less protected rather than more. The skeleton receives fewer mechanical signals, the muscles weaken further, and confidence continues to shrink.

That is why this section needs to stay focused on the relationship rather than treating bone and muscle as different chapters of ageing. A person with osteoporosis does not only need concern about fracture risk. They need as much muscle support, balance support, and movement confidence as possible. And a person losing muscle should not assume that bone is unaffected by that decline. In many cases, bone and muscle are deteriorating within the same broader pattern of reduced loading, reduced reserve, and increasing vulnerability.

In practical terms, the message is clear: preserving muscle helps protect more than muscle. It helps support the body that carries the skeleton. It helps reduce the likelihood of the fall that becomes the fracture. It helps keep movement more stable, more confident, and less fearful. When muscle is maintained well, bone health is not guaranteed, but the body is often in a far better position than when muscle and bone are both being left to drift downward together.

That is why osteoporosis belongs in this chapter. It reminds the reader that chronic conditions do not usually isolate themselves neatly. They overlap, and the overlap matters. A stronger body is often a safer body. And when bone becomes more fragile, the need for muscle preservation becomes even more urgent, not less.

Cardiovascular Disease and Reduced Physical Reserve

Cardiovascular disease changes more than the heart. It changes the amount of physical reserve a person has available for everyday life. This is one reason it belongs in a chapter about muscle loss. When cardiovascular health declines, people often do less, tire sooner, recover more slowly, and become more vulnerable to deconditioning. Over time, those changes can make muscle harder to preserve even if muscle was not the original clinical focus. Sarcopenia is increasingly recognised as common in cardiovascular disease and associated with faster disease progression, higher mortality, falls, and reduced quality of life.

This matters because cardiovascular disease and muscle decline often reinforce each other. A weaker, less active body has less physical reserve to support circulation, glucose control, function, and recovery. At the same time, symptoms such as fatigue, breathlessness, lower exercise tolerance, and fear of overexertion can reduce activity enough that muscle begins to decline more quickly. The result is not simply heart disease on one side and muscle loss on the other. It is a body becoming less capable across multiple connected systems.

For many readers, the lived experience of this is not dramatic at first. It may begin as walking less because hills feel harder, avoiding stairs because recovery takes longer, or losing confidence in exercise because the body no longer responds with the same steadiness it once did. That gradual reduction in physical demand matters. As discussed throughout this book, muscle is maintained when it is repeatedly asked to stay. If cardiovascular symptoms steadily lower the amount of effort the body has to produce, muscle often becomes one of the tissues that quietly pays the price.

There is also an emotional side to this that should not be ignored. People living with cardiovascular disease often become more cautious around exertion, and sometimes with good reason. But caution can slowly turn into underuse if everything physically demanding begins to feel risky. Once that happens, the body may become less conditioned, less strong, and less tolerant of effort, which then reinforces the fear that exertion is unsafe. This is one reason reduced physical reserve can be so self-reinforcing. The person is not only dealing with disease. They are dealing with a shrinking sense of what their body can still handle.

This section also needs to make clear that cardiovascular disease does not make muscle preservation irrelevant. It makes it more important. The evidence suggests that sarcopenia is not only more common in people with cardiovascular disease, but that worsening sarcopenia status is associated with higher future cardiovascular risk, while recovery from sarcopenia is associated with lower risk. That is an encouraging point because it means decline is not the only direction that matters. Improvement matters too.

In practical terms, the key issue is not whether a person with cardiovascular disease can train as if nothing has changed. Often they cannot, and that needs respect. The key issue is whether the body can still be given enough safe, appropriate stimulus to protect muscle, movement, and confidence. If not, physical reserve tends to narrow further. If so, the person is often in a better position not only to preserve muscle, but to cope with the broader demands of chronic disease. That is why this section belongs in the chapter. Cardiovascular disease is not only a circulatory problem. It is often a reserve problem, and muscle is one of the main places that loss of reserve becomes visible.

Chronic Inflammatory Conditions and Accelerated Muscle Loss

Chronic inflammation changes the environment in which muscle is trying to survive. This is one reason inflammatory conditions belong in a chapter on accelerated muscle loss. The issue is not only that a person has a diagnosed disease. It is that persistent inflammatory activity can make the body less supportive of muscle maintenance, less responsive to exercise, less efficient in recovery, and often less able to sustain normal physical activity over time.

This matters because inflammation does not act on muscle in isolation. It often arrives alongside fatigue, pain, appetite disruption, poorer sleep, lower movement confidence, and periods of reduced activity. Over time, those pressures begin to overlap. A person may move less because they feel unwell, eat less because appetite is poor, recover less effectively because the body is already under strain, and gradually lose strength because the conditions needed to preserve muscle are no longer as reliable as they once were. The muscle loss is not random. It is part of a body that is being pulled in a more catabolic direction.

This helps explain why chronic inflammatory conditions can accelerate decline even when they do not seem primarily "muscular." A person may think of the problem as bowel disease, autoimmune disease, chronic inflammatory illness, or another systemic condition, while the muscle changes happen more quietly in the background. But those changes matter. If inflammation remains elevated and physical reserve is not actively protected, muscle often becomes one of the tissues that steadily loses ground.

There is also a practical side to this that readers may recognise immediately. Chronic inflammatory conditions often make life less predictable. Some days are manageable. Other days feel heavier, more painful, more exhausting, or less stable. That unpredictability can make routine harder to maintain. Exercise becomes more stop-start. Meals may become less consistent. Recovery may feel incomplete. The body can start to feel like something that has to be constantly negotiated rather than trusted. Under those conditions, muscle preservation becomes harder not only because of biology, but because the rhythm of life becomes harder to sustain.

This is one reason inflammation should not be thought of only as a laboratory issue or something that matters only to doctors. For the reader, its real importance is that it changes how the body feels and functions. It can make movement more costly, effort less rewarding, and recovery less reliable. If those changes continue long enough, physical reserve begins to narrow. The person may not notice it immediately as "muscle loss," but it shows up in reduced strength, less stamina, slower recovery, lower confidence, and a growing sense that the body is becoming less cooperative.

At the same time, this section should not suggest that chronic inflammatory conditions make muscle decline unavoidable. They increase vulnerability, but they do not erase the value of intervention. In many cases, preserving muscle becomes even more important because the body is under more strain. Resistance training may need adaptation. Daily movement may need to be protected more intentionally. Protein intake may need more attention, especially when appetite is inconsistent. Recovery may need more respect. But the core principle remains the same: the body still benefits from being given a reason to stay strong.

There is a deeper emotional burden here too. Chronic inflammatory illness can make people feel as though they are losing control of their body in unpredictable waves. That can lead to a kind of physical resignation, where the person stops expecting stability and begins to lower their demands of themselves. Sometimes that caution is necessary. But if it becomes a long-term withdrawal from challenge, the body often becomes less resilient rather than more protected. This is why preserving muscle in the presence of chronic inflammation is not just about tissue. It is also about resisting the slow narrowing of life that can follow repeated illness, fatigue, and uncertainty.

In practical terms, the most important message is that inflammation makes muscle preservation more urgent, not less relevant. A body under chronic inflammatory pressure has more reason to lose muscle, which means it has more reason to be supported deliberately. The strategy may need to be more flexible, more patient, and more responsive to fluctuations, but the goal remains the same: protect as much strength, function, and independence as possible even when health is not straightforward.

Mitochondria and Energy Production in Diseased Muscle

Muscle is one of the most energy-demanding tissues in the body. Every contraction, every effort to stand, lift, climb, recover, and adapt depends on a constant supply of usable energy. This is where mitochondria matter. Mitochondria are the structures inside muscle cells that help produce that energy, and skeletal muscle contains them in abundance because it relies so heavily on continuous metabolic work.

This matters because chronic disease often affects muscle not only through inflammation, inactivity, or poor nutrition, but also through energy production itself. When mitochondrial function becomes less efficient, muscle may become more fatigue-prone, less resilient, and less able to respond well to physical demand. A person may notice this not as a laboratory finding, but as something much more familiar: the body feels less steady, less responsive, and less capable of sustaining effort than it once did.

That is one reason mitochondria deserve a place in this chapter. They help explain why diseased muscle often struggles more even when the problem does not appear, on the surface, to be a "muscle disease." In conditions such as type 2 diabetes, obesity, cardiovascular disease, and chronic inflammatory illness, muscle is often operating in a less favourable energy environment. It may be receiving poorer metabolic signals, carrying more oxidative stress, or functioning with less efficient cellular machinery. Over time, this can help explain why the body feels more easily drained and why maintaining muscle becomes harder under chronic health strain.

This is also one reason fatigue should not be dismissed as a vague or purely motivational issue. Sometimes a person living with chronic disease feels that their body no longer produces energy in a reliable way. Effort feels more expensive. Recovery feels less complete. Physical work that once felt ordinary now leaves a deeper mark. These experiences are not only psychological. They may reflect a body whose energy systems are under greater strain.

At the same time, this section should not make mitochondria sound mysterious or detached from daily life. Their importance becomes practical when you understand what they support. They help muscle keep producing force, keep tolerating movement, and keep adapting to training. When mitochondrial function declines, the body may find it harder to preserve muscle quality, physical stamina, and metabolic resilience. That is why diseased muscle often feels less forgiving. It is not only carrying more biological stress. It is often doing so with less efficient energy support.

There is also an encouraging side to this. Mitochondrial health is not entirely fixed. Movement, resistance training, and a more supportive nutritional environment can all help create conditions in which muscle functions more effectively. This does not mean chronic disease disappears or that mitochondria become a miracle explanation for everything. It means muscle remains responsive even at the level of its energy machinery, which is one more reason preserving movement and strength still matters when health is complicated.

In practical terms, this section deepens the chapter's main message. Chronic disease accelerates muscle loss not only by making people move less or eat less well, but by making muscle itself less efficient and less resilient. Mitochondria help explain that part of the story. They remind the reader that when disease makes the body feel more tired, slower to recover, and less physically reliable, muscle is often struggling at the energy level as well as the mechanical one.

That is why mitochondria belong here. They help connect the conditions in this chapter into one clearer picture: diseased muscle often has to work harder under worse conditions. And the more that picture is understood, the easier it becomes to see why preserving muscle remains one of the most protective strategies available.

Medication Considerations

Medication needs to be handled carefully in a chapter like this because the goal is not to make you suspicious of treatment. The goal is to help you understand that medication effects can sometimes influence muscle preservation indirectly, and occasionally directly, without implying that medicines should be stopped casually or feared by default. In most cases, the right message is not to avoid medication. It is to see the whole picture. Polypharmacy in older adults has been associated with weaker muscle, poorer physical performance, and slower functional recovery, but the practical response is thoughtful review and muscle-protective planning, not alarm.

This matters because medications can affect the same daily realities discussed throughout this book. They may influence your appetite, energy, dizziness, sleep, balance, gastrointestinal comfort, or willingness to move. Even when a drug is appropriate and important, you may still find that training feels harder, meals feel less appealing, or recovery feels less predictable. In those cases, the issue is not whether the medication is good or bad. The issue is whether your muscle-preservation plan is taking those effects into account.

This becomes especially relevant in older age because the number of medications often increases as health becomes more complex. The more layered treatment becomes, the more likely it is that small effects on fatigue, steadiness, appetite, or exercise tolerance begin to matter in practical life. You may not notice one major problem. Instead, you may notice that you feel slightly less steady, slightly less hungry, slightly more tired, or slightly less willing to challenge your body. Those small shifts can matter over time because they affect the consistency of training, movement, and intake.

That is why medication review belongs in a muscle-preservation chapter. It is not here to tell you to stop treatment on your own. It is here to remind you that if strength is falling, appetite is worsening, fatigue is rising, or movement confidence is dropping, medication burden may be one part of the discussion worth reviewing with your doctor or pharmacist. In practical terms, this means asking better questions. Is this medicine affecting your appetite? Does it make activity harder? Could timing, dose, or the overall medication mix be contributing to falls, dizziness, poor intake, or low energy? Those are sensible questions. They are not anti-medication questions.

Statins are a good example of why this section needs balance. They are often discussed in public conversation as though they automatically damage muscle, but current review level evidence does not support a simple conclusion that statin exposure increases sarcopenia risk in older adults. At the same time, some people do experience muscle symptoms while taking them, and those symptoms deserve proper assessment rather than dismissal. The careful message is that symptoms should be evaluated, not assumed, and that proven cardiovascular benefits should not be casually undermined by oversimplified fear.

There is also an emotional side to this. If you are already managing chronic disease, you are probably carrying enough uncertainty as it is. You do not need to become afraid of every prescription. But it does help to understand that medication lives inside a wider physical system. If your body feels less capable, less hungry, less steady, or more tired, it is reasonable to consider whether treatment burden is part of the overall picture. That awareness can make your conversation with a clinician more useful and more grounded.

In practical terms, the safest and most useful takeaway is this: medications are often necessary and beneficial, but they should be viewed in context. Muscle preservation works best when treatment, training, nutrition, and recovery are considered together rather than separately. You do not need to become fearful of medication. You need to become more informed about how to protect muscle while living with the realities that treatment sometimes brings.

Protecting Muscle in the Presence of Chronic Disease

If you are living with chronic disease, the most important thing to understand is that muscle preservation still matters. In many ways, it matters more. When health becomes more complicated, your body needs more physical reserve, not less. You need strength to tolerate interruptions, recover after illness, stay steady when energy is lower, and keep doing ordinary tasks when life is not running smoothly. Chronic disease may change the conditions in which your body operates, but it does not remove the value of protecting muscle. It makes that protection more urgent.

This is one of the most important messages in the chapter because it is easy to fall into the belief that muscle can wait until the "real" health issues are sorted out first. But muscle is not separate from those issues. It is part of how you cope with them. It helps support glucose control, movement, balance, bone loading, physical confidence, and the ability to recover from setbacks. The stronger and more capable your body remains, the more reserve you have when chronic disease places extra strain on the system.

That does not mean the approach should be rigid. It means it should be realistic. If you are living with pain, fatigue, medication effects, inflammatory flares, poor appetite, or variable exercise tolerance, then your muscle-preservation strategy has to be built around those realities rather than pretending they do not exist. Training may need to be smaller, more flexible, or more carefully paced. Nutrition may need more intention because appetite is unreliable. Recovery may need more respect because the body is carrying more physiological load. But none of those changes mean the plan has lost value. They mean the plan has become more intelligent.

This is where people often underestimate the power of consistency. You may not be able to train at the level you once did. You may not always feel energetic. You may need to work around symptoms, appointments, treatment schedules, painful days, or health events that interrupt routine. But even then, a body that keeps receiving some signal to stay strong is usually better protected than a body that is repeatedly left to decondition. The goal is not perfection under perfect circumstances. The goal is continuity under real circumstances.

There is also a deeper emotional truth here. Chronic disease can make you feel as though your body is becoming more medical than physical, more something to manage than something to trust. When that happens, strength work, movement, and good nutrition can start to feel secondary. But they are not secondary. They are part of how you keep your body from becoming smaller, weaker, and less confident than it needs to be. They are part of how you stay involved in your own life rather than gradually withdrawing from it.

This is why the practical foundations of muscle preservation still matter so much. Keep resistance training in your life in some form, even if it has to be adapted. Keep daily movement as part of your routine, even if the amount changes from week to week. Keep protein and overall intake supported as well as your appetite and health status allow. Keep recovery in the picture instead of treating fatigue and sleep as irrelevant background issues. These are not glamorous strategies, but they are often the ones that protect the most function over time.

You also need to be willing to work with your body instead of against it. Some days will require more adjustment than others. Some periods will allow progress, while others will call for maintenance. Sometimes protecting muscle means pushing a little. Sometimes it means simplifying without disappearing. The skill is in knowing that both can still be part of forward movement.

In practical terms, chronic disease does not cancel the muscle-preservation story. It changes the terrain, but not the destination. You are still trying to protect strength, function, resilience, and independence. The path may be less straightforward, but the goal remains just as important. In many cases, it is one of the most useful things you can still work toward.

Conclusion

Chronic disease does not affect muscle by accident. It affects muscle because it changes the conditions that muscle depends on. It can reduce movement, increase inflammation, impair recovery, disrupt appetite, alter energy handling, and make the body less efficient at preserving strength and function over time. That is why conditions such as type 2 diabetes, obesity, osteoporosis, cardiovascular disease, chronic inflammatory illness, and treatment burden so often appear alongside muscle decline. They do not just coexist with it. They often help drive it.

This matters because muscle is one of the main forms of protection you carry when health becomes more complicated. It helps support glucose control, steadiness, bone loading, physical confidence, movement capacity, and the ability to recover after illness or interruption. When muscle declines in the setting of chronic disease, the loss is rarely limited to appearance or gym performance. It shows up in the practical parts of life: lower tolerance, slower recovery, poorer resilience, greater fatigue, and a body that feels less reliable than it once did.

One of the most important ideas in this chapter is that chronic disease should not push muscle preservation to the side.

It should move it closer to the centre. The more strain your body is under, the more valuable physical reserve becomes. The more complicated your health picture is, the more important it is to protect the tissue that helps you keep functioning within it. That does not mean the strategy will always be simple. It may require more flexibility, more patience, and more careful adjustment. But it is still worth doing.

This chapter has also shown that the drivers of muscle loss in chronic disease are not all visible from the outside. Some are mechanical. Some are metabolic. Some are inflammatory. Some involve energy production at the cellular level. Some relate to medications, appetite, or lower activity tolerance. Together, they explain why diseased muscle often struggles more and why preserving it requires a more deliberate approach than many people expect.

The encouraging message is that none of this makes muscle preservation irrelevant. It makes it more practical. You may not be able to remove every disease burden, medication effect, inflammatory pressure, or fatigue constraint. But you can still work to preserve as much strength, movement, and physical confidence as possible within those realities. That work matters because it helps keep the body more capable under conditions that would otherwise make decline easier.

If there is one practical takeaway from this chapter, it is this: chronic disease may accelerate muscle loss, but protecting muscle remains one of the most useful ways to protect yourself. It helps support function, resilience, and independence not in spite of complicated health, but because health is complicated. That is exactly why it matters.

Chapter 14: Putting It All Together: A Lifelong Muscle Preservation Framework

Introduction

By this point in the book, one message should be clear: muscle preservation is never the result of one isolated choice. It is not created by protein alone, training alone, or recovery alone. It is shaped by the way these factors work together over time. That is why a final chapter like this matters. Without integration, it is easy to understand the parts of muscle preservation while still struggling to see how they fit together in real life.

This matters because the body does not experience life in separate chapters. It does not divide training from nutrition, sleep from appetite, inflammation from recovery, or chronic disease from movement capacity. These factors overlap constantly. A person who trains well but eats poorly is not getting the same result as someone who supports both. A person who eats enough protein but sleeps badly, moves little, and carries a high inflammatory burden is not living in the same physical environment as someone whose recovery is better supported. A person with chronic disease or pain does not step outside the muscle-preservation story. They are living inside it under more difficult conditions.

That is why the most useful way to understand lifelong muscle preservation is as a system. Some parts of that system matter more directly than others. Some act as primary drivers, while others shape how well those primary drivers can work. But all of them influence the same outcome: whether your body remains strong, resilient, and physically capable across time.

This chapter brings those pieces together. Its job is not to repeat every earlier chapter in condensed form. Its job is to help you think more clearly. It should leave you with a way of making decisions when life is normal, when life is busy, when health is complicated, and when the body is no longer behaving ideally. In that sense, this chapter is less about new information and more about usable order. It asks not only what matters, but what matters most first.

That distinction is important because many people lose traction not through lack of effort, but through lack of hierarchy. They worry about supplements while neglecting training. They focus on meal details while chronically under-eating protein. They become interested in gut health while remaining sedentary. They become discouraged by pain, illness, or poor sleep and assume the whole system has failed. What they often need is not more complexity. They need a clearer sense of priority.

There is also something reassuring in thinking this way. It means muscle preservation does not depend on doing everything perfectly at once. It depends on understanding the system well enough to protect its strongest levers first, then improve the conditions around them as life allows. That is a much more realistic and sustainable way to approach the body, especially across different life stages and changing health conditions.

This is also why the framework in this chapter needs to stay practical. It should help you understand what to emphasise when you are younger and building reserve, when you are in midlife protecting it, when you are older and trying to preserve independence, and when pain, illness, fatigue, or chronic disease make the path less straightforward. The principles remain connected, but their emphasis changes depending on what your body most needs at the time.

Seen clearly, lifelong muscle preservation is not a collection of tricks. It is a way of managing physical capacity across changing circumstances. The rest of this chapter is built to make that idea usable. It begins with the framework itself.

The Lifelong Muscle Preservation Framework

A useful muscle-preservation framework begins with a simple truth: not everything matters equally at the same level. Some factors are primary. They create the main stimulus that tells the body to keep muscle, maintain function, and protect physical reserve. Other factors are modifiers. They shape how well the primary signals are received, supported, and sustained. Both matter, but they do not matter in the same order.

The primary levers are resistance training, adequate protein intake, and enough daily movement to stop the body from slipping into habitual underuse. These are the clearest signals you can give your body that muscle is still needed. Resistance training tells the body that strength matters. Protein helps provide the building material and anabolic support required to maintain and repair tissue. Daily movement helps preserve the broader physical environment in which muscle remains functionally relevant rather than biologically expensive and easy to lose.

These primary levers deserve to be placed first because without them, the rest of the system has little to work with. You can optimise recovery perfectly, but if you never challenge the body, muscle has less reason to stay. You can improve diet quality in general, but if protein remains too low, one of the main nutritional supports for muscle is still missing. You can care deeply about inflammation, sleep, or gut health, but if the body lives in chronic underuse, muscle is still being told that it is not especially necessary.

That does not make the secondary factors unimportant. It makes them secondary in role, not in value. Sleep, stress regulation, diet quality, inflammatory load, gut health, clinical stability, and medication awareness all influence how well the primary levers can work. They affect how well you recover, how strongly you adapt, how stable your appetite is, how efficient your metabolism remains, and how much resilience your body has when life becomes more difficult. These factors often explain why two people with similar training habits can get very different results over time.

A clear framework therefore works in layers. First, you protect the main levers. Then you improve the conditions around them. Then you adapt both of those layers to the life stage and health context you are living in. That sequence matters because it helps prevent distraction. It keeps you from chasing advanced details while neglecting the fundamentals that matter more. In practical terms, this means asking three levels of question.

First: are you giving your body enough reason to keep muscle at all? Are you training with resistance in some meaningful form? Are you eating enough protein often enough? Are you moving enough day to day that the body still experiences itself as physically needed?

Second: are you creating a recovery and nutritional environment that helps those signals work well? Are you sleeping enough for recovery to occur? Is your diet pattern supportive rather than inflammatory and erratic? Are you carrying chronic stress, fatigue, under-eating, or low-grade illness burden that may be blunting adaptation? Is your gut environment being supported through sound whole-diet quality rather than hype and fragmentation?

Third: what is your current life stage and constraint profile? Are you building reserve, protecting reserve, preserving independence, or adapting around pain, disease, or interrupted recovery? The answer changes the emphasis of the plan, even when the core logic stays the same.

This layered approach is one of the most useful ways to simplify the complexity of muscle preservation. It allows you to stop treating every factor as equally urgent. It helps you see that the system has structure. The body needs the main signals first. Then it benefits from improved conditions around those signals. Then the whole plan must be shaped around the realities of age, health, pain, illness, and imperfect life circumstances.

There is also an emotional benefit to this framework. It reduces the sense that you must do everything at once or that one imperfect area makes the whole effort pointless. If sleep is not ideal, the primary levers still matter. If pain is present, some training signal can often still be protected. If chronic disease complicates things, protein, movement, and recovery still deserve attention. The framework helps you keep thinking clearly when life is not neat.

That is why this chapter is ending the book with a system rather than a list. Lists are easy to forget. Systems are easier to return to. When you understand the order of importance, you are less likely to be pulled off course by trends, fear, or discouragement. You begin to see that lifelong muscle preservation is not about mastering endless details. It is about protecting the strongest drivers of physical capacity and then supporting them intelligently over time.

The Primary Levers: Resistance Training, Protein, and Daily Movement

If you want to protect muscle across the lifespan, these are the levers that deserve the most attention first: resistance training, adequate protein, and enough daily movement to prevent the body from slipping into habitual underuse. They are not the whole story, but they are the strongest controllable drivers in it. If these are neglected, the rest of the system has much less to build on.

Resistance training comes first because it provides the clearest direct signal that muscle is still needed. It asks the body to produce force, maintain tissue, preserve function, and keep physical reserve available for real-life demands. Across earlier adulthood, midlife, and older age, resistance training remains one of the most reliable ways to protect strength, maintain lean tissue, and support independence. The form may change across the lifespan, but the basic principle does not. If you ask your muscles to stay useful, they are far more likely to remain so.

Protein sits beside training because muscle is not preserved by stimulus alone. It also needs support. Resistance training creates the demand for adaptation, but protein helps provide the raw material and anabolic environment required for repair, retention, and rebuilding. That is why the earlier chapters on protein mattered so much. The point was never that protein acts in isolation. It was that without enough of it, one of the body's main muscle-supportive resources is weakened. Training and protein are not competitors. They are partners.

Daily movement matters because your body is responding to more than formal exercise sessions. It is also responding to the broader rhythm of how physically engaged your life is. A person who resistance trains a few times a week but otherwise lives in prolonged underuse is still giving the body mixed signals. Daily movement helps preserve coordination, metabolic health, circulation, joint confidence, and general physical demand. It may not replace resistance training, but it makes the whole environment more supportive of muscle preservation rather than less.

This is one reason these levers must be treated as primary. They are the factors that most directly answer the question, "Why should the body keep this muscle?" Resistance training says the muscle is needed for force and function. Protein says the body has enough nutritional support to help maintain it. Daily movement says physical usefulness is still part of everyday life rather than something switched on only occasionally. Together, these signals create a far stronger case for preserving muscle than any isolated strategy on its own.

There is also something deeply practical about this. Many people get pulled toward more complicated concerns before they have protected these fundamentals. They worry about supplements, nutrient timing, gut-health products, advanced recovery methods, or other fine details while undertraining, under-eating protein, or remaining too sedentary. That does not mean the finer details are meaningless. It means they work best when the main levers are already in place. The fundamentals are not exciting because they are simple. They are powerful because they keep working.

These primary levers also travel well across life stages. In earlier adulthood, they help build reserve. In midlife, they help protect reserve against drift, disuse, and competing demands. In older age, they help preserve independence, steadiness, and functional capacity. In chronic disease, they become part of how the body continues to cope with health burdens without surrendering more strength than necessary. The emphasis changes, but the core logic remains consistent.

There is an emotional benefit to seeing these as primary too. It simplifies the path. If your life is busy or your health is not ideal, you do not need to solve every variable before making progress. You need to ask whether these main levers are being protected strongly enough. Are you giving your body a reason to stay strong? Are you feeding it in a way that supports that goal? Are you moving enough that physical capacity still feels relevant to daily life? Those are grounding questions. They keep you focused on what matters most when everything else feels noisy.

In practical terms, if you are unsure where to begin, begin here. Strengthen your body in some repeatable way. Support it with enough protein. Keep it moving across the day. These three levers will not solve every problem, but they create the strongest foundation on which the rest of the system can work. Without them, muscle preservation becomes much harder than it needs to be. With them, the rest of the framework becomes far more effective and far more meaningful.

The Secondary Modifiers: Recovery, Sleep, Stress, Gut Health, and Inflammation

Once the primary levers are in place, the next question is how well your body is positioned to respond to them. This is where the secondary modifiers matter. They do not replace resistance training, protein, or daily movement, but they strongly influence how effective those primary signals become. In other words, they help determine whether your body is working in a more supportive environment or a more resistant one.

Recovery sits near the top of this layer because adaptation does not happen during effort alone. It happens in the period that follows it. If your sleep is poor, your stress load is high, your appetite is unstable, or your body is carrying a high inflammatory burden, the same training and nutrition inputs may produce less benefit than they otherwise would. This is one reason some people feel as though they are doing many of the right things but still struggling to move forward. The main levers may be present, but the environment around them is making adaptation harder.

Sleep matters here because it influences muscle protein synthesis, hormonal balance, appetite regulation, recovery capacity, and training responsiveness. As discussed earlier in this book, poor sleep does not merely make you tired. It can change the biology through which muscle is maintained and recovered. That does not mean every bad night undoes your progress. It means chronic poor sleep can quietly reduce how well your body responds to the other things you are trying to do right.

Stress matters for similar reasons. A body under persistent stress is not functioning in the same way as one that is recovering well. Chronic stress can alter cortisol regulation, appetite, inflammation, sleep quality, and recovery behaviour. It can also change how willing you are to train, how well you tolerate effort, and how consistently you eat and move. This is why stress should not be thought of as something separate from muscle preservation. It becomes part of the environment in which your body is either adapting or struggling to adapt.

Gut health belongs in this layer too, but carefully. It is not a magic shortcut, and it should not be treated as more important than the primary levers. But it does matter because the gut helps shape inflammation, nutrient handling, and the broader internal environment in which muscle is maintained. A supportive dietary pattern, fibre intake, and a healthier gut environment may improve the conditions around muscle preservation, even if they do not replace the need for training and protein. This is why gut health makes sense as a modifier rather than a main driver.

Inflammation is one of the clearest modifiers of all because it can blunt adaptation across several pathways at once. Chronic low-grade inflammation can interfere with anabolic signalling, worsen fatigue, reduce recovery efficiency, and make the body less responsive to exercise and nutrition. This does not mean you can eliminate inflammation completely or that every inflammatory influence is under your control. It means that diet quality, sleep, movement, metabolic health, and disease management all matter partly because they influence whether your body is operating in a more inflamed or more supportive state.

This layered view is important because it helps you think more clearly when progress feels uneven. If the main levers are present but results are weaker than expected, the next place to look is often not a more advanced supplement or a more complicated program. It is the modifiers. Are you sleeping enough to recover? Is stress constantly raising the cost of effort?

Is your diet quality supporting or worsening inflammatory load? Is your gut environment likely helping or hindering nutrient handling and immune balance? These questions make more sense once the primary levers are already being protected.

There is also a practical comfort in understanding this order. It means you do not need to obsess over secondary factors before the fundamentals are in place. But it also means that once the fundamentals are in place, improving the environment around them can make a real difference. That is the role of modifiers. They are not the engine of muscle preservation, but they can make the engine run better or worse.

In practical terms, this section should leave you with a simple understanding: train, eat enough protein, and keep moving first. Then ask whether sleep, stress, gut health, and inflammation are helping those efforts work well or quietly getting in their way. That is how the system stays clear. The main levers come first. The modifiers determine how much support those levers receive once they are already in motion.

Adapting the Framework Across Life Stages

The framework in this chapter stays consistent across life, but the emphasis does not. That is one of the most important ways to make it useful. Resistance training, adequate protein, daily movement, recovery, diet quality, and health context matter throughout the lifespan, but they do not carry the same urgency in exactly the same way at every stage. What changes is not the foundation. What changes is what your body most needs from that foundation at the time.

In earlier adulthood, the priority is building reserve. This is the stage where the body is generally more responsive, recovery is often easier, and there is more opportunity to build strength, muscle, and physical confidence from a higher baseline. At this point, the framework is less about rescuing decline and more about accumulation. The primary levers still come first, but their purpose is to establish as much useful reserve as possible before life becomes more physically and metabolically demanding. This is why earlier adulthood matters so much. It is not just a stage of fitness. It is a stage of preparation.

In midlife, the emphasis shifts from building reserve to protecting it. This is often the period when competing demands begin to pull people away from the habits that once kept them stronger and more resilient. Work becomes more sedentary. Recovery is less forgiving. Training is easier to interrupt. Appetite, sleep, and body composition may begin to drift in unhelpful directions. This is the stage where the framework becomes protective in a more deliberate way. The body may still feel broadly capable, but the cost of neglect starts to rise. That is why midlife is such an important turning point. It is often the stage when the body stops rewarding autopilot.

In older age, the emphasis shifts again. Now the goal is not just preserving reserve in the abstract, but protecting independence directly. Strength still matters, but power and balance become more urgent because they help determine how safely and confidently you move through daily life. Nutrition becomes more intentional because appetite may be less reliable. Recovery becomes more important because illness, poor sleep, and interruptions can take a greater toll. The framework still works the same way, but the meaning becomes more visible. It is no longer only about preserving future protection. It is about preserving present function.

Chronic disease changes the framework in a different way. It does not replace life stage, but it changes the terrain at any stage. A person living with type 2 diabetes, obesity, cardiovascular disease, inflammatory illness, pain, medication burden, or reduced energy availability is working within a body that may be less efficient, more inflamed, less resilient, or more fatigue-prone. In that setting, the same framework still applies, but it has to be adapted more carefully. The primary levers still matter. In many ways, they matter more. But the modifiers and constraints become more influential, which means the plan often has to become more flexible, more patient, and more realistic.

This is why a lifelong framework is better than a one-size-fits-all prescription. It allows the same core logic to travel across changing circumstances without pretending that all circumstances are the same. You do not need a completely different philosophy for each decade. You need a consistent framework with changing emphasis. Build reserve earlier. Protect it through midlife. Preserve independence later. Adapt intelligently when illness, pain, or chronic disease make the path less straightforward.

There is also something reassuring in that continuity. It means you are not starting from scratch every time life changes. You are still working with the same main levers. You are still trying to preserve strength, function, and physical reserve. What changes is the way you prioritise and apply them. That gives the framework both stability and flexibility, which is exactly what a useful long-term system needs.

In practical terms, this section should leave you with a simple understanding: the framework does not need to be reinvented at every stage of life. It needs to be re-weighted. The core principles stay connected. The emphasis shifts with age, recovery capacity, health complexity, and functional need. That is what makes the system lifelong rather than temporary.

What to Do When Life Is Not Ideal

No one lives inside a perfect muscle-preservation environment for very long. Illness happens. Pain flares. Sleep worsens. Appetite drops. Work gets heavy. Stress becomes chronic. Travel interrupts routine. Motivation falls. Energy becomes unreliable. If your framework only works when life is smooth, it is not a very useful framework. A lifelong system has to work under ordinary, imperfect conditions, not just under ideal ones. That is one reason the final chapter has to address this directly. The best framework is not the one that looks most complete on paper. It is the one you can keep using when life becomes less cooperative.

This matters because imperfect periods are often where people lose the most ground. Not always because the setback itself is severe, but because the whole system collapses at once. Training stops. Meals become erratic. Protein falls. Movement drops. Sleep worsens. The body then receives fewer reasons to stay strong at exactly the time it is already under more strain. Over time, this pattern can do far more damage than the difficult week, painful flare, or stressful month that started it. That is why the question during imperfect periods should never be whether everything can still be done perfectly. The question is what must be protected first.

The answer usually begins with the primary levers. If life is difficult, protect some version of resistance training, some version of adequate protein, and some version of daily movement before worrying about finer details. A shorter session still counts. A reduced training week still counts. Simpler meals with meaningful protein still count. Walking more gently still counts. These are not lesser efforts in a dismissive sense. They are the forms of effort that keep the system alive when ideal conditions are gone. The body is still listening for the same message: am I still needed, and am I still being supported?

This becomes especially important during pain, arthritis, tendon flare-ups, and interrupted training. As discussed earlier in the book, the danger is rarely just the painful event itself. The larger danger is the stop-start pattern that follows when every setback turns into full disengagement. If life is not ideal, the more useful response is often not to stop everything, but to scale intelligently. Reduce load. Change exercise selection. Shorten the session. Shift the emphasis. Keep a signal alive. That is how the body retains more readiness, and that is often how confidence survives as well.

Low appetite and fatigue need the same kind of realism. There will be periods when eating well feels harder than it should. In older age especially, appetite may become less reliable at exactly the stage when nutritional support matters more. During those periods, the aim is not dietary perfection. The aim is to stop nutritional drift from becoming prolonged under-support. Simpler meals may be necessary. Repeated foods may be necessary. Convenience may need to become more strategic. What matters is that muscle is not quietly starved of support while the body is already dealing with illness, recovery pressure, or low energy.

Poor sleep and high stress require the same calm hierarchy. They matter, and they can strongly blunt recovery, appetite regulation, and training responsiveness. But they do not automatically mean progress is impossible. What they do mean is that expectations may need to shift for a period. The goal may move from progress to maintenance, from full training to minimum effective dose, or from optimisation to continuity. This is where people often go wrong. They assume that because conditions are not good enough for ideal progress, the whole effort has become pointless. In reality, maintenance during difficult periods is often one of the most valuable forms of progress available.

There is also an emotional truth here that the framework should acknowledge clearly. When life is not ideal, you may feel as though your body is slipping out of reach. You may feel behind, discouraged, or tired of having to adapt. You may feel as though everyone else is operating under simpler conditions. This is exactly when the framework needs to become more useful, not less. Its job is not to shame you for imperfection. Its job is to help you decide what matters most when you cannot do everything. That is where hierarchy becomes powerful. You do not need to solve every problem at once. You need to stop the system from going dark.

In practical terms, when life is not ideal, think in this order. Keep some training signal alive. Keep protein support as intact as possible. Keep moving more than complete withdrawal would suggest. Then improve sleep, stress, diet quality, and recovery as conditions allow. This order matters because it stops difficult periods from turning into full-body drift. It keeps the strongest levers active while allowing the modifiers to be improved more gradually rather than all at once.

Seen clearly, imperfect weeks are not failures of the framework. They are where the framework proves whether it is real. If it can guide you through illness, pain, poor sleep, low appetite, interrupted routine, and difficult seasons without losing sight of what matters most, then it is a useful lifelong system. And that is exactly what this one is meant to be.

A Decision-Making System for Real Life

A framework becomes truly useful when it helps you decide what to do next, not just what matters in theory. That is the purpose of this section. When life becomes busy, recovery worsens, pain flares, appetite drops, or chronic disease complicates the picture, you need a way to think clearly about priority. You need a system that helps you ask not, "How do I optimise everything at once?" but, "What matters most right now?" That is where the lifelong muscle-preservation framework becomes most practical.

The first question is always the same: are the primary levers still active? Are you doing some form of resistance training? Are you getting enough protein to support muscle? Are you moving enough day to day that your body is still being told it is physically needed? If the answer is no, those are the first things to address. Not perfectly, but clearly. When the primary levers are missing, it makes little sense to become overly focused on more refined issues before those foundations are back in place.

If the primary levers are present but progress still feels limited, the next question is whether the modifiers are getting in the way. Are you sleeping poorly enough that recovery is being blunted? Is chronic stress changing your appetite, motivation, or tolerance for effort? Is your diet quality making inflammation and recovery worse rather than better? Are pain, illness, gut issues, or treatment burden creating a body that is harder to support than it appears from the outside? This is where the framework becomes more nuanced. It helps you stop assuming you need more complexity when what you may actually need is a better recovery and health environment around the fundamentals.

If your main problem is undertraining, the answer is not usually a supplement or a more detailed nutrition plan. It is to restore some consistent mechanical demand. If your main problem is under-eating protein, the answer is not a more advanced training split. It is to improve the nutritional support your muscle is receiving. If your main problem is poor recovery, then forcing harder training on top of sleep debt, illness, or high stress may simply increase frustration. In each case, the framework helps you return to the real bottleneck instead of chasing whatever seems most interesting in the moment.

If you are in earlier adulthood, the decision-making system should keep asking whether you are building reserve strongly enough. If you are in midlife, it should ask whether you are protecting reserve against drift, underuse, and rising recovery cost. If you are in older age, it should ask whether your current choices are protecting independence, power, balance, appetite support, and physical confidence. If you are living with chronic disease, it should ask whether the framework is being adapted to your reality rather than abandoned because the terrain is harder. The same system works, but the emphasis changes depending on where you are and what your body is currently facing.

This is also where imperfect weeks need to be handled differently from failed weeks. If life is difficult, the question becomes: what is the minimum I need to preserve so the system does not go dark? That may mean keeping one or two resistance sessions, protecting protein even with simpler meals, walking more than complete withdrawal would suggest, or reducing training volume without letting the habit disappear. Maintenance during difficult periods is often the most intelligent form of progress available, because it preserves the body's readiness for when conditions improve.

A useful way to think about the system is this. If strength is declining, first check whether you are training enough to justify keeping it. If training is in place, check whether protein support is too low. If both are in place, check whether sleep, stress, illness, inflammation, or health burden are blunting the response. If pain or chronic disease is part of the picture, ask how the plan needs to be adapted rather than whether it should be abandoned. That order matters because it stops you from solving the wrong problem first.

There is also an emotional benefit to having a system like this. It reduces confusion. It helps stop discouragement from turning into drift. When things are not working, you do not have to assume the whole effort is failing. You can assess which part of the system is weakest and strengthen that first. That makes the process calmer, more deliberate, and far more sustainable across the changing conditions of real life.

In practical terms, this is the decision-making sequence: protect the primary levers first, improve the modifiers second, adapt the emphasis to your life stage and constraints, and during difficult periods, preserve the minimum that keeps the system alive.

That is the lifelong muscle-preservation framework at its most useful. It is not only a way of understanding the body. It is a way of deciding what to do next when the body, your schedule, or your health are not making the answer obvious.

Conclusion

If this book has one central message, it is this: muscle is not a luxury tissue. It is one of the main foundations of physical independence, metabolic stability, resilience, and healthy ageing. It helps you move, recover, cope with illness, tolerate stress, protect bone, regulate glucose, and stay capable in the ordinary tasks that make up a life. When muscle is preserved well, the body usually carries more reserve. When it is neglected, the consequences are rarely confined to strength alone.

That is why muscle preservation should never be reduced to appearance, gym culture, or the pursuit of a younger body. It is about function. It is about whether your body remains reliable enough to carry you through the decades ahead. It is about whether ageing becomes a gradual narrowing of physical capacity or a process you meet with as much reserve as possible still intact.

Throughout this book, you have seen that muscle is shaped by more than one influence. Training matters. Protein matters. Diet quality matters. Recovery matters. Gut health, inflammation, clinical conditions, pain, appetite, stress, and sleep all matter too. But the deeper lesson is not that everything matters equally. It is that muscle preservation becomes far more manageable when you understand the order of importance. Protect the main levers first. Support the environment around them second. Adapt the strategy to your age, your health, and your real-life constraints rather than waiting for ideal conditions that may never come.

That way of thinking changes the whole task. It means you do not need perfection to make progress. You do not need to solve every weakness at once. You do not need a body free of pain, disease, interruption, or fatigue before your efforts become worthwhile. You need a clear enough framework to keep protecting what matters most, even when life is difficult. That is how long-term strength is preserved. Not by flawless execution, but by continued intelligent effort.

There is also something hopeful in this. The body remains responsive for longer than many people assume. Muscle can still be built, protected, and meaningfully supported across the lifespan. It may become harder to maintain when recovery is poorer, when health is more complicated, or when life is more crowded. But harder does not mean pointless. In many cases, it means more important.

If you are younger, the message is to build reserve before you need it. If you are in midlife, the message is to protect reserve before decline becomes harder to reverse. If you are older, the message is to preserve independence, power, and confidence for as long as possible. If you are living with pain, illness, chronic disease, or imperfect conditions, the message is not that you are excluded from the muscle-preservation story. It is that your strategy may need to be more adaptive, but it remains deeply worth pursuing.

So if there is one final practical takeaway from this book, let it be this: do not wait until strength feels urgent before you begin treating it as important. Protect muscle early. Protect it consistently. Protect it intelligently. The return on that effort is not only measured in muscle itself. It is measured in freedom, steadiness, resilience, and the ability to keep living inside your body with confidence for as long as possible.

That is what lifelong muscle preservation is really about.

Glossary

Actin
A contractile protein in muscle fibres that works with myosin to produce force.

Adaptive response
The body's ability to improve or adjust after a stimulus such as training, protein intake, or recovery.

Anabolic
Refers to processes that build or repair tissue, including muscle.

Anabolic resistance
A reduced ability of ageing muscle to respond to protein intake and exercise with a strong muscle-building or muscle-preserving response.

Amino acids
The building blocks of protein. Some are especially important for repairing and maintaining muscle tissue.

Anorexia of ageing
A decline in appetite that often occurs in older age, making it harder to eat enough to maintain health and muscle.

ATP (adenosine triphosphate)
The main energy source your cells use for muscle contraction and many other body processes.

Body composition
The relative amounts of muscle, fat, bone, and other tissues in the body.

Catabolic
Refers to processes that break tissue down, including muscle breakdown.

Chronic low-grade inflammation
A persistent, mild inflammatory state that can interfere with recovery, metabolic health, and muscle maintenance over time.

Connective tissue
Supportive tissue that helps hold structures together. In muscle, this includes the layers that surround fibres and help transmit force.

Cortisol
A hormone involved in stress response, energy regulation, and recovery. It is necessary in normal amounts, but chronically elevated levels can work against muscle preservation.

Cross-bridge cycle
The microscopic process in which myosin binds to actin and generates force during muscle contraction.

Energy availability
The amount of energy left for normal body function after the energy cost of exercise has been accounted for.

Essential amino acids
Amino acids that the body cannot make on its own and must obtain from food.

Fascicle
A bundle of muscle fibres grouped together within a muscle.

Fast-twitch fibres
Muscle fibres that produce force quickly and powerfully but fatigue faster. They are important for speed, power, and rapid balance recovery.

Frailty
A state of reduced physical reserve and increased vulnerability to stressors such as illness, falls, or hospitalisation.

Glycaemic control
How well the body keeps blood glucose within a healthy range.

Glycogen
The stored form of carbohydrate in muscle and liver, used as a major fuel source during exercise.

Growth hormone
A hormone involved in tissue repair, body composition, and recovery. Its secretion is closely linked to sleep, especially deep sleep.

Gut–muscle axis
The relationship between gut health, inflammation, nutrient handling, and muscle health.

Hypertrophy
An increase in muscle fibre size, usually in response to resistance training and adequate nutrition.

IGF-1 (insulin-like growth factor-1)
A hormone involved in growth, tissue repair, and muscle adaptation.

Inflammaging
The chronic low-grade inflammation often associated with ageing, which can contribute to muscle decline and reduced recovery capacity.

Insulin sensitivity
How effectively the body responds to insulin. Better insulin sensitivity helps muscles take up and use glucose more effectively.

Leucine
An essential amino acid that plays an important role in stimulating muscle protein synthesis.

Mechanical loading
Physical stress placed on muscles and bones through activity or exercise, especially resistance training.

Metabolic health
The health of systems involved in blood glucose control, energy use, fat storage, and related functions.

Mitochondria
Structures inside cells that help produce energy. Because muscle needs a lot of energy, mitochondrial health strongly affects muscle function and recovery.

Motor neuron
A nerve cell that sends signals from the nervous system to muscle fibres, telling them to contract.

Motor unit
A motor neuron and all the muscle fibres it controls.

mTOR
A major signalling pathway involved in regulating muscle protein synthesis and growth.

Muscle mass
The total amount of muscle tissue in the body.

Muscle protein breakdown
The process of breaking down muscle proteins. This happens normally, but it becomes a problem when it regularly exceeds rebuilding.

Muscle protein synthesis
The process of building new muscle proteins. This is stimulated by protein intake and resistance exercise.

Muscle quality
How well muscle functions relative to its size. A muscle can look large enough but still perform poorly if quality is reduced.

Myofibril
A thread-like structure inside a muscle fibre containing the contractile machinery of the muscle.

Myokines
Signalling molecules released by muscle that can affect inflammation, metabolism, and other body systems.

Myosin
A contractile protein that interacts with actin to create muscle contraction.

Myosteatosis
Fat accumulation within or around muscle tissue that reduces muscle quality and function.

Neuromuscular
Relating to both nerves and muscles, especially how the nervous system controls muscle function.

Oxidative stress
A state where damaging reactive molecules build up faster than the body can neutralise them, potentially affecting cells and tissues.

Phosphagen system
The fastest energy system in the body, used for short, explosive efforts such as lifting heavy weights or sprinting.

Physical reserve
The extra strength, function, and resilience your body has available beyond basic daily needs.

Power
The ability to produce force quickly. In ageing, power is especially important for preventing falls and maintaining independence.

Progressive resistance training
Resistance training that gradually becomes more challenging over time so the body continues to adapt.

Protein distribution
How protein is spread across meals during the day, rather than consumed mainly in one meal.

Protein turnover
The continuous cycle of muscle protein breakdown and muscle protein synthesis.

Recovery capacity
How well your body can repair, adapt, and return to function after stress such as training, illness, or poor sleep.

Relative Energy Deficiency in Sport (RED-S)
A condition caused by chronically low energy availability that disrupts recovery, hormones, performance, and health.

Resistance training
Exercise that challenges muscles against a load, such as weights, bands, machines, or body weight.

Sarcopenia
Age-related loss of muscle mass, strength, and function.

Sarcopenic obesity
A condition in which excess body fat exists alongside low muscle mass, low strength, or poor muscle quality.

Satellite cells
Muscle stem cells involved in repair, regeneration, and adaptation after damage or training.

Sarcolemma
The outer membrane of a muscle fibre.

Sarcomere
The smallest functional unit of muscle contraction inside a muscle fibre.

Short-chain fatty acids
Compounds produced when gut bacteria ferment fibre. They may help influence gut health, inflammation, and metabolism.

Slow-twitch fibres
Muscle fibres that are more fatigue-resistant and better suited to endurance and postural tasks.

Slow-wave sleep
Deep sleep, important for restoration, hormonal regulation, and recovery.

Strength
The ability to produce force.

Systemic inflammation
Inflammation that affects the body more broadly rather than being limited to one local area.

Tendon
A tough connective tissue structure that attaches muscle to bone and helps transmit force.

Type I fibres
Another name for slow-twitch muscle fibres.

Type II fibres
Another name for fast-twitch muscle fibres.

Ultra-processed foods
Industrially formulated foods often made from refined ingredients and additives. When they dominate the diet, they can weaken overall diet quality.

Visceral adiposity
Fat stored deep around the abdominal organs, often linked with inflammation and metabolic dysfunction.

References

Affourtit, C., & Carré, J. E. (2024). Mitochondrial involvement in sarcopenia. Acta Physiologica, 240, e14107.

Agarwal, V., Baranwal, M., Gandhi, M., Pal, A., Navik, U., & Nair, A. K. (2025). Elucidating the potential mechanism and therapeutic strategies of chronic stress-induced skeletal muscle atrophy. Life Sciences, 379, 123615.

Androulakis-Korakakis, P., Fisher, J. P., & Steele, J. (2020). The minimum effective training dose required to increase 1RM strength in resistance-trained men: A systematic review and meta-analysis. Sports Medicine, 50(4), 751–765.

Ans, A. H., Anjum, I., Satija, V., et al. (2018). Neurohormonal regulation of appetite and its relationship with stress: A mini literature review. Cureus, 10(7), e3032.

Artigas-Arias, M., Alegría-Molina, A., Fernández-Lázaro, D., Gutiérrez-Abejón, E., García-Gómez, A., & Mielgo-Ayuso, J. (2024). Skeletal muscle mass, strength, and physical performance gains are similar between healthy postmenopausal women and postmenopausal breast cancer survivors after 12 weeks of resistance exercise training. Sports, 12(11), 295.

Asano, Y., Yoshida, T., Tsunoda, K., Yokoyama, K., Watanabe, Y., Yoshinaka, Y., Okura, T., Kimura, M., & Yamada, Y. (2025). Sex- and age-related declines in muscle mass, strength, physical performance, and muscle quality among community-dwelling older adults: A cross-sectional study. Experimental Gerontology, 210, 112862.

Atherton, P. J., & Smith, K. (2012). Muscle protein synthesis in response to nutrition and exercise. The Journal of Physiology, 590(5), 1049–1057.

Australian Institute of Health and Welfare. (2024). Insufficient physical activity. Australian Institute of Health and Welfare.

Balachandran, A. T., Steele, J., Angulo, J., Giangregorio, L. M., Rose, D. J., & Seguin, R. C. (2022). Power training vs traditional strength training for physical function in older adults: A systematic review and meta-analysis. JAMA Network Open, 5(5), e2211623.

Barry, D. J., Wu, S. S. X., & Cooke, M. B. (2025). The relationship between gut microbiota, muscle mass and physical function in older individuals: A systematic review. Nutrients, 17(1), 81.

Baskurt, H. P., Esen, G., Karabudak, E., Kiziltan, G., Hocaoglu, M. B., & Rakicioglu, N. (2025). Consumption of ultra-processed foods can accelerate age-related sarcopenia. Nutrients, 17(12), 2057.

Bauer, J., et al. (2013). Evidence-based recommendations for optimal dietary protein intake in older people: A position paper from the PROT-AGE Study Group. Journal of the American Medical Directors Association, 14(8), 542–559.

Beaudart, C., et al. (2014). The effects of vitamin D on skeletal muscle strength, muscle mass, and muscle power: A systematic review and meta-analysis. Journal of Clinical Endocrinology & Metabolism, 99(11), 4336–4345.

Besora-Moreno, M., Llauradó, E., Tarro, L., Solà, R., & Moreira-Rosário, A. (2024). Effects of probiotics, prebiotics, and synbiotics on sarcopenia-related outcomes in older adults: A systematic review. Journal of Cachexia, Sarcopenia and Muscle, 15(6), 2470–2483.

Bloom, I., Shand, C., Cooper, C., Robinson, S., & Baird, J. (2018). Diet quality and sarcopenia in older adults: A systematic review. Nutrients, 10(3), 308.

Borba, V. Z. C., Costa, T. L. M., de Camargo Cánova, J., Boguszewski, C. L., & Moreira, C. A. (2025). Sarcopenic obesity: A review. Archives of Endocrinology and Metabolism, 69(2), e230198.

Bouchonville, M. F., & Villareal, D. T. (2013). Sarcopenic obesity: How do we treat it? Current Opinion in Endocrinology, Diabetes and Obesity, 20(5), 412–419.

Breen, L., & Phillips, S. M. (2011). Skeletal muscle protein metabolism in the elderly: Interventions to counteract the 'anabolic resistance' of ageing. Nutrition & Metabolism, 8(1), 68.

Briand, M., Dekeuleneer, M., Gielen, E., et al. (2025). Body composition and aging: Cross-sectional results from the SarcoAge study. GeroScience, 47, 2357–2371.

Brooks, G. A. (2018). The science and translation of lactate shuttle theory. Cell Metabolism, 27(4), 757–785.

Broome, S. C., Whitfield, J., Karagounis, L. G., & Hawley, J. A. (2024). Mitochondria as nutritional targets to maintain muscle health and physical function during ageing. Sports Medicine, 54(9), 2291–2309.

Buendía-Romero, Á., Alegre, L. M., & Aguado-Jiménez, R. (2025). Residual effects of physical exercise after periods of training cessation in older adults: A systematic review. International Journal of Environmental Research and Public Health, 22(1), 414.

Bull, F. C., et al. (2020). World Health Organization 2020 guidelines on physical activity and sedentary behaviour. British Journal of Sports Medicine, 54(24), 1451–1462.

Campbell, W. W., Bales, C. W., Beasley, J. M., & Evans, M. (2023). Nutritional interventions: Dietary protein needs and influences on skeletal muscle of older adults. Current Opinion in Clinical Nutrition and Metabolic Care, 26(4), 241–248.

Cappellari, G. G., Chiappetta, S., & Muttini, S. (2024). Detecting sarcopenia in obesity: Emerging new approaches. Current Opinion in Clinical Nutrition and Metabolic Care, 27(5), 321–327.

Caturano, A., Amaro, A., Galiero, R., Pafundi, P. C., Rinaldi, L., Salvatore, T., Cesaro, A., Moscarella, E., Gragnano, F., Sasso, F. C., & Marfella, R. (2025). Sarcopenic obesity and weight loss-induced muscle mass loss. Current Opinion in Clinical Nutrition and Metabolic Care, 28(4), 201–208.

Chang, A. H., Lee, J., Song, J., et al. (2025). Temporal associations of physical activity with subsequent pain in adults with chronic musculoskeletal conditions. Pain Reports, 10(2), e1217.

Cheng, M., Wang, X., Li, Y., et al. (2025). Optimal type and dose of exercise to improve fall-related outcomes in older adults: A systematic review and network meta-analysis. Maturitas, 195, 108352.

Chilibeck, P. D., Kaviani, M., Candow, D. G., & Zello, G. A. (2017). Effect of creatine supplementation during resistance training on lean tissue mass and muscular strength in older adults: A meta-analysis. Open Access Journal of Sports Medicine, 8, 213–226.

Choi, S., Chon, J., Kim, H.-S., Lee, S. A., Lee, Y., Lim, J.-Y., & Won, C. W. (2023). Impact of vitamin B12 insufficiency on the incidence of sarcopenia and its components in older adults. Nutrients, 15(4), 936.

Choi, S., Park, J., Kim, H., et al. (2025). Effects of resistance exercise programs on strength and functional performance in older adults: A systematic review. Journal of Exercise Rehabilitation, 21(1), 12–25.

Choudhary, P. K., Sharma, R., Singh, N., et al. (2025). Effectiveness of balance- and strength-based exercise interventions in older adults: A systematic review and meta-analysis. BMC Geriatrics, 25, 114.

Claudino, J. G., et al. (2021). Strength training to prevent falls in older adults: Systematic review and meta-analysis of RCTs. Journal of Clinical Medicine.

Clifford, C., Challoumas, D., Paul, L., Syme, G., & Millar, N. L. (2020). Effectiveness of isometric exercise in the management of tendinopathy: A systematic review and meta-analysis of randomised trials. BMJ Open Sport & Exercise Medicine, 6(1), e000760.

Coelho-Junior, H. J., Rodrigues, B., Uchida, M., & Marzetti, E. (2022). Protein intake and sarcopenia in older adults: A systematic review and meta-analysis. Nutrients, 14(8), 1632.

Copinschi, G. (2013). Sleep and hormonal changes in aging. Endocrinology and Metabolism Clinics of North America, 42(2), 371–389.

Cornish, S. M., Myrie, S. B., Bugera, E. M., Chase, J. E., Turczyn, D., & Pinder, M. A. (2022). Effects of omega-3 supplementation alone and combined with resistance exercise on skeletal muscle in older adults: A systematic review and meta-analysis. Nutrients, 14(11), 2221.

Cruz-Jentoft, A. J., et al. (2019). Sarcopenia: Revised European consensus on definition and diagnosis. Age and Ageing, 48(1), 16–31.

Currier, B. S., et al. (2023). Resistance training prescriptions and outcomes: Bayesian network meta-analysis. British Journal of Sports Medicine.

Dalle, S., Rossmeislova, L., & Koppo, K. (2017). The role of inflammation in age-related sarcopenia. Frontiers in Physiology, 8, 1045.

Daly, R. M., Bollen, C., Bollen, J., et al. (2024). Sarcopenia in general practice: Towards improving muscle health screening, assessment and management in Australia. Australian Journal of General Practice, 53(10), 751–755.

Damluji, A. A., Forman, D. E., van Diepen, S., Alexander, K. P., Brawner, C. A., Cleveland, J. C., Jr., Givertz, M. M., Hummel, S. L., Keteyian, S. J., Link, M. S., Rich, M. W., Rodriguez, F., & Zieman, S. J. (2023). Sarcopenia and cardiovascular diseases. Circulation, 147(20), 1537–1553.

Dattilo, M., Antunes, H. K. M., Medeiros, A., et al. (2011). Sleep and muscle recovery: Endocrinological and molecular basis for a new and promising hypothesis. Medical Hypotheses, 77(2), 220–222.

Deane, C. S., Wilkinson, D. J., Phillips, B. E., & Smith, K. (2024). Critical variables regulating age-related anabolic resistance to exercise and nutrition. Frontiers in Nutrition, 11, 1419229.

Deutz, N. E. P., et al. (2014). Protein intake and exercise for optimal muscle function with aging: Recommendations from the ESPEN Expert Group. Clinical Nutrition.

Devries, M. C., & Phillips, S. M. (2014). Creatine supplementation during resistance training in older adults: A meta-analysis. Medicine & Science in Sports & Exercise, 46(6), 1194–1203.

Dharap, V., Govani, S. M., Liu, J., et al. (2025). Prevalence and outcome of sarcopenia in patients with inflammatory bowel disease. Intestinal Research, 23(1), 77–86.

Di Lorito, C., Long, A., Byrne, A., Harwood, R. H., Gladman, J. R. F., Schneider, S., Logan, P., Bosco, A., & van der Wardt, V. (2021). Exercise interventions for older adults: A systematic review of meta-analyses. Journal of Sport and Health Science, 10(1), 29–47.

Dias, R. K. N., Gama, D. R. N., Nunes, J. P., et al. (2024). Minimal-dose resistance training enhances muscle strength and functional capacity in older adults. Scientific Reports, 14, 69073.

Donini, L. M., et al. (2022). Definition and diagnostic criteria for sarcopenic obesity: ESPEN and EASO consensus statement. Obesity Facts.

Duchateau, J., et al. (2021). Strength training: In search of optimal strategies. Exercise and Sport Sciences Reviews.

Dyer, S. M., et al. (2023). Exercise for falls prevention in residential aged care: Systematic review and meta-analysis. Age and Ageing.

Dáttilo, M., Antunes, H. K. M., Galbes, N. M., et al. (2020). Effects of sleep deprivation on acute skeletal muscle recovery after exercise-induced muscle damage in young men. Sleep and Biological Rhythms, 18, 145–152.

Feng, Z., Zhang, Y., Zhang, X., et al. (2025). A systematic review and meta-analysis of biomarker mechanisms in sarcopenia and sarcopenic obesity. International Journal of Molecular Sciences, 26(11), 5113.

Fernandes, L., Santos, R., Oliveira, A., et al. (2025). Effects of strength training on the quality of life of older adults: A systematic review. Geriatrics, 5(4), 49.

Fisher, J. P., Steele, J., Gentil, P., Giessing, J., & Westcott, W. L. (2017). A minimal dose approach to resistance training for the older adult: The prophylactic for aging. Experimental Gerontology, 99, 80–86.

Fragala, M. S., Cadore, E. L., Dorgo, S., et al. (2019). Resistance training for older adults: Position statement from the National Strength and Conditioning Association. Journal of Strength and Conditioning Research, 33(8), 2019–2052.

Frampton, J., Murphy, K. G., Frost, G., & Chambers, E. S. (2021). Higher dietary fibre intake is associated with increased skeletal muscle mass and strength in adults aged 40 years and older. Journal of Cachexia, Sarcopenia and Muscle, 12(6), 2134–2144.

Garcia, J. M., & Merriam, G. R. (2019). Growth hormone and aging. In K. R. Feingold, B. Anawalt, A. Boyce, et al. (Eds.), Endotext. MDText.com, Inc.

Georgiou, G. D., Saunders, B., Bampouras, T. M., et al. (2024). Effect of beta-alanine supplementation on maximal intensity exercise in trained young male individuals: A systematic review and meta-analysis. International Journal of Sport Nutrition and Exercise Metabolism, 34(6), 397–409.

Gomez, R. J., Martinez, L. P., & Santos, D. A. (2025). Mitigation of detraining effects: Physical activity improves recovery after detraining in older adults. Experimental Gerontology, 188, 112401.

Gong, H., Cheng, M., Chen, Y., Qin, Y., Zhu, Y., Li, M., & Duan, Y. (2025). Association between dietary index for gut microbiota and sarcopenia: Mediation by inflammatory dietary burden. Frontiers in Nutrition, 12, 1569950.

Grgic, J., Grubic, T., Pickering, C., Del Coso, J., Schoenfeld, B. J., & Mikulic, P. (2021). Effects of caffeine on resistance exercise: A review of recent evidence. Sports Medicine, 51(11), 2281–2298.

Hall, J. E. (2021). Guyton and Hall textbook of medical physiology (14th ed.). Elsevier.

Hallajzadeh, J., Tanha, K., Khatibi, S. R., Clark, C. C. T., & Moradi, S. (2025). The impact of ultra-processed food consumption on frailty and sarcopenia: A systematic review. Ageing Research Reviews, 106, 102771.

Hamidvand, A., et al. (2025). Acute effects of resistance exercise on skeletal muscle glycogen: Systematic review with meta-analysis. Physiology Reports.

Handajani, Y. S., Noor, N., Wangko, S., Tjandrawinata, R. R., & Santoso, A. (2024). Probiotic supplementation or probiotic-fortified products on sarcopenic indices in older adults: A systematic review and meta-analysis. Nutrition Reviews, 82(7), 837–854.

Harris, S., Barnes, T., Chew, J., & Isenring, E. (2025). Protein and aging: Practicalities and practice. Nutrients, 17(15), 2461.

Hojjati Kermani, M. A., Awlqadr, F. H., Talebi, S., Mehrabani, S., Ghoreishy, S. M., Wong, A., Mohammadi, H., Clark, C. C. T., & Moradi, S. (2025). The association of ultra-processed food intake on age-related muscle conditions: A systematic review and dose-response meta-analysis with meta-regression. Journal of Health, Population and Nutrition, 44, 271.

Houston, D. K., et al. (2023). Vitamin D supplementation and muscle power/strength/physical performance. The American Journal of Clinical Nutrition.

Huang, N., Ge, M., Bi, X., et al. (2025). A framework of biomarkers for skeletal muscle aging: A consensus statement by the Aging Biomarker Consortium. Ageing Research Reviews, 103, 102632.

Huang, Y., Wang, C., Cui, H., Sun, G., Qi, X., & Yao, X. (2025). Mitochondrial dysfunction in age-related sarcopenia: Mechanistic insights, diagnostic advances, and therapeutic prospects. Frontiers in Cell and Developmental Biology, 13, 1590524.

Hudson, J. L., Bergia, R. E., & Campbell, W. W. (2020). Protein distribution and muscle-related outcomes: Does the evidence support the concept? Nutrients, 12(5), 1441.

Hurst, C., et al. (2022). Resistance exercise as a treatment for sarcopenia. Age and Ageing.

Ibrahim, K., Walker, T., Mach, J., et al. (2025). The evidence and impact of deprescribing on sarcopenia parameters in older adults: A systematic review. BMC Geriatrics, 25, 581.

Ispoglou, T., McCullough, D., & Norton, C. (2025). Editorial: Preventing sarcopenia and promoting musculoskeletal health in middle-aged adults: The role of exercise and nutrition. Frontiers in Nutrition, 12, 1597800.

Janssen, T. A. H., Lowisz, C. V., & Phillips, S. M. (2025). From molecular to physical function: The aging trajectory. Current Research in Physiology, 8, 100138.

Jeong, I., Cho, E. J., Yook, J. S., Choi, Y., Park, D. H., Kang, J. H., Lee, S. H., Seo, D. Y., Jung, S. J., & Kwak, H. B. (2024). Mitochondrial adaptations in aging skeletal muscle: Implications for resistance exercise training to treat sarcopenia. Life, 14(8), 962.

Jiang, G., Liu, Y., Wang, X., et al. (2025). A 24-week combined resistance and balance training program improves physical function in older adults. Journal of Strength and Conditioning Research, 39(1), 188–197.

Jiménez-Lupión, D., Ramírez-Campillo, R., et al. (2023). Power training and functional capacity related to fall risk in older adults: A systematic review and meta-analysis. Experimental Gerontology, 176, 112169.

Jin, S., Li, C., Huang, R., et al. (2025). The correlation between sarcopenia and osteoporosis in older adults: A systematic review and meta-analysis. Osteoporosis International, 36, 1123–1135.

Judelson, D. A., et al. (2007). Does fluid balance affect strength, power and high-intensity endurance? Sports Medicine.

Kaji, H. (2025). Bone-muscle interactions. Osteoporosis and Sarcopenia, 11(2), 78–86.

Kamarulzaman, N. T., & Makpol, S. (2025). The link between mitochondria and sarcopenia. Journal of Physiology and Biochemistry, 81(1), 1–20.

Kasicki, K., Kaczmarczyk, M., & Wójcik, A. (2025). Multicomponent versus single-component exercise interventions in older adults: A systematic review and meta-analysis. BMC Geriatrics, 25, 603.

Katsuhara, S., Yokomoto-Umakoshi, M., Umakoshi, H., et al. (2022). Impact of cortisol on reduction in muscle strength and mass: A Mendelian randomization study. The Journal of Clinical Endocrinology & Metabolism, 107(4), e1477–e1487.

Kenney, W. L., Wilmore, J. H., & Costill, D. L. (2020). Physiology of sport and exercise (7th ed.). Human Kinetics.

Khodadad Kashi, S., Mirzazadeh, Z. S., & Saatchian, V. (2023). A systematic review and meta-analysis of resistance training on quality of life, depression, muscle strength, and functional exercise capacity in older adults aged 60 years or more. Biological Research for Nursing, 25(1), 88–106.

Kiehl, D., Kittelson, A. J., Christiansen, C. L., et al. (2025). Relationship of lifetime strength training exposure with knee pain and physical function in adults at risk of osteoarthritis. Journal of Exercise Science & Fitness, 23(2), 145–153.

Kim, B., Osuka, Y., Okubo, Y., Zhao, X., Kim, G.-M., & Oh, S. (2025). The physical activity paradox in low muscle mass in middle-aged and older adults. American Journal of Preventive Medicine, 68(2), 348–356.

Kim, H., Kim, J., Lee, C., & Kim, S. (2025). Nutrition and exercise for sarcopenia treatment. Osteoporosis and Sarcopenia, 11(2 Suppl), 54–64.

Kitagawa, T., Sato, Y., Nakamura, M., et al. (2025). Effectiveness of exercise therapy in patients with knee osteoarthritis: An overview of systematic reviews. BMC Musculoskeletal Disorders, 26, 771.

Kjær, B. H., Madsen, C. G., Juul-Kristensen, B., et al. (2024). To allow or avoid pain during shoulder rehabilitation exercises in chronic rotator cuff-related shoulder pain? A randomized controlled trial. Musculoskeletal Science and Practice, 69, 102870.

Kokura, Y., et al. (2024). Enhanced protein intake on maintaining muscle mass in adults with overweight/obesity aiming for weight loss. Clinical Nutrition ESPEN.

Kumar, R., Dewan, A., & Sharma, S. (2025). Sarcopenia and diabetes in older adults in the decade of healthy aging: A comprehensive review. Archives of Gerontology and Geriatrics, 131, 105802.

Kunz, H. E., O'Reilly, E. L., Harris, M. M., et al. (2023). Age-associated inflammation and implications for skeletal muscle health and exercise adaptation. Experimental Gerontology, 175, 112145.

Lamon, S., Morabito, A., Arentson-Lantz, E., et al. (2021). The effect of acute sleep deprivation on skeletal muscle protein synthesis and the hormonal environment. Physiological Reports, 9(1), e14660.

Lapauw, L., Descamps, B., Maes, K., De Buyser, S., De Cock, A.-M., Gielen, E., Vandewoude, M., & Goossens, G. H. (2024). Associations between gut microbiota and sarcopenia or its defining parameters in older adults: A systematic review. Journal of Cachexia, Sarcopenia and Muscle, 15(5), 1937–1954.

Lapauw, L., Descamps, B., Maes, K., De Buyser, S., De Cock, A.-M., Gielen, E., Vandewoude, M., & Goossens, G. H. (2025). Effect of host- and gut microbiota-altering interventions on sarcopenia parameters: A systematic review. Ageing Research Reviews, 105, 102718.

Larsson, L., Degens, H., Li, M., Salviati, L., Lee, Y. I., Thompson, W., Kirkland, J. L., & Sandri, M. (2019). Sarcopenia: Aging-related loss of muscle mass and function. Physiological Reviews, 99(1), 427–511.

Lee, E., Kim, J., & Park, S. (2025). Physical activity and protein-intake strategies to prevent sarcopenia in older adults. International Health, 17(4), 423–432.

Leitão, L., Silva-Reis, M., Ribeiro, A., et al. (2024). Detraining and retraining effects of a multicomponent exercise program on physical function in older adults. European Review of Aging and Physical Activity, 21, 7.

Li, J., Vitiello, M. V., & Gooneratne, N. S. (2018). Sleep in normal aging. Sleep Medicine Clinics, 13(1), 1–11.

Li, S., Liu, J., Chen, X., Zhang, Y., Wang, Y., & Zhao, L. (2025). Association of dietary index for gut microbiota and sarcopenia in adults: A cross-sectional analysis. Nutrition & Metabolism, 22, 118.

Li, W., Zheng, Y., Wang, D., Zhang, X., & Zhang, Y. (2024). Exploring the relationship between gut microbiota and sarcopenia. Nutrients, 16(21), 3691.

Li, X., Wang, B., Liu, L., et al. (2023). Sleep duration and sarcopenia: An updated systematic review and meta-analysis. Journal of the American Medical Directors Association, 24(8), 1193–1201.e3.

Liang, Z., Wu, X., Cheng, Y., et al. (2022). Inflammaging: The ground for sarcopenia? Frontiers in Cell and Developmental Biology, 10, 970241.

Liguori, S., et al. (2024). Role of magnesium in skeletal muscle health. International Journal of Molecular Sciences.

Lim, J., Park, H., Lee, S., et al. (2024). The effects of resistance training on pain, strength, and function in knee and hip osteoarthritis: A systematic review and meta-analysis. Sports Medicine - Open, 10, 96.

Liu, C. J., & Latham, N. K. (2009). Progressive resistance strength training for improving physical function in older adults. Cochrane Database of Systematic Reviews.

Liu, Y., Chen, H., Zhang, P., Shang, Q., Zhang, Y., Qiu, W., Zhang, Y., He, J., Zhao, W., Qin, W., Lin, F., Ren, H., Jiang, X., & Shen, G. (2025). The additive effect of sarcopenia and osteoporosis on all-cause mortality: A cohort analysis in a U.S. population. Scientific Reports, 15, 43408. https://doi.org/10.1038/s41598-025-00003-8

Longland, T. M., Oikawa, S. Y., Mitchell, C. J., Devries, M. C., & Phillips, S. M. (2016). Higher compared with lower dietary protein during an energy deficit combined with intense exercise promotes greater lean mass retention. The American Journal of Clinical Nutrition.

Luo, J., Lee, R. Y. W., & Chen, T. (2025). Physical activity reduces the incidence of sarcopenia in middle-aged adults. Ageing International, 50, 1–12.

Mamerow, M. M., et al. (2014). Dietary protein distribution positively influences 24-h muscle protein synthesis in healthy adults. The Journal of Nutrition.

Marzetti, E., Calvani, R., Lorenzi, M., et al. (2025). Defective mitochondrial quality control in the aging of skeletal muscle. Mechanisms of Ageing and Development, 229, 112019.

Mata, F., et al. (2019). Carbohydrate availability and physical performance: Physiological basis and practical implications. Nutrients.

Matos, A., Tihon, C., Costa, C., & Domingues, C. (2025). Current strategies for healthy aging: The interplay between nutrition, metabolism, and exercise. Cureus, 17(11), e96848.

Mayer, M. H., Woldemariam, S., Gisinger, C., Lamprecht, M., & Tschan, H. (2024). Association of gut microbiome with muscle mass, muscle strength, and muscle performance in older adults: A systematic review. International Journal of Environmental Research and Public Health, 21(9), 1246.

McArdle, W. D., Katch, F. I., & Katch, V. L. (2015). Exercise physiology: Nutrition, energy, and human performance (8th ed.). Lippincott Williams & Wilkins.

McClure, R., Villani, A., & Kellett, J. (2017). Mediterranean diet attenuates risk of frailty and sarcopenia: New insights and future directions. JCSM Clinical Reports, 2(2), 1–17.

McGregor, R. A., Cameron-Smith, D., & Poppitt, S. D. (2014). It is not just muscle mass: A review of muscle quality, composition and metabolism during ageing. Ageing Research Reviews, 18, 45–58.

McKendry, J., Morton, J. P., & Breen, L. (2024). Mitigating disuse-induced skeletal muscle atrophy in ageing: Resistance exercise as a critical countermeasure. Experimental Physiology, 109(10), 1904–1917.

Merry, K., Docking, S., Rio, E., & Cook, J. (2024). Perspectives of people with Achilles tendinopathy and physical therapists on tendon loading and pain: A qualitative survey study. BMJ Open Sport & Exercise Medicine, 10(1), e001724.

Mitchell, W. K., Williams, J., Atherton, P., Larvin, M., Lund, J., & Narici, M. (2012). Sarcopenia, dynapenia, and the impact of advancing age on human skeletal muscle size and strength. Journal of Cachexia, Sarcopenia and Muscle, 3(4), 260–269.

Mocini, E., Cardinali, L., Di Vincenzo, O., Moretti, A., de Sire, A., de Sire, R., & Migliaccio, S. (2025). An integrated nutritional and physical activity approach for osteosarcopenia. Nutrients, 17(17), 2842.

Mondéjar-Barrios, M. D., Garcia-Esquinas, E., Ortolá, R., et al. (2026). Effect of statin use on the development of sarcopenia in older adults: A systematic review and meta-analysis. Drugs & Aging, 43(2), 115–128.

Moon, G. K., & Bu, S. Y. (2023). Effects of omega-3 fatty acid supplementation on skeletal muscle mass and strength in adults: A systematic review. Clinical Nutrition Research, 12(4), 304–318.

Morgan, E., Irwin, M. R., Chung, M., et al. (2017). Sleep characteristics and daytime cortisol levels in older adults. Sleep, 40(11), zsx128.

Morton, R. W., et al. (2018). A systematic review, meta-analysis and meta-regression of protein supplementation on resistance training-induced gains in muscle mass and strength. British Journal of Sports Medicine, 52(6), 376–384.

Morton, R. W., et al. (2018). Protein supplementation and resistance training-induced gains in muscle mass and strength: Systematic review, meta-analysis and meta-regression. British Journal of Sports Medicine, 52(6), 376–384.

Moss, C., & Dhillo, W. S. (2012). The regulation of appetite and the anorexia of ageing. Current Opinion in Clinical Nutrition and Metabolic Care, 15(1), 21–25.

Mountjoy, M., et al. (2023). 2023 International Olympic Committee (IOC) consensus statement on Relative Energy Deficiency in Sport (RED-S). British Journal of Sports Medicine, 57(17), 1073–1097.

Murphy, C., Koehler, K., & others. (2022). Energy deficiency impairs resistance training gains in lean mass but not strength: A meta-analysis and meta-regression. Scandinavian Journal of Medicine & Science in Sports.

Murray, B., & Rosenbloom, C. (2018). Fundamentals of glycogen metabolism for coaches and athletes. Nutrition Reviews, 76(4), 243–259.

Nayab, S., Khan, S., Ali, R., et al. (2024). The impact of exercise interventions on pain, function, and quality of life in knee osteoarthritis: A systematic review and meta-analysis. BMC Musculoskeletal Disorders, 25, 1008.

Nowakowska-Lipiec, K., Maciejczyk, M., Niestrój-Jaworska, M., et al. (2025). Progressive loss of muscle strength: The effects of ageing and sarcopenia on muscle function in older females. Journal of Clinical Medicine, 14(20), 7276.

Nuzzo, J. L. (2024). Resistance exercise minimal dose strategies for increasing strength: A narrative review. Sports Medicine, 54(8), 1749–1765.

Pana, A., Sourtzi, P., Kalokairinou, A., et al. (2021). Association between muscle strength and sleep quality and duration among middle-aged and older adults: A systematic review. Aging Clinical and Experimental Research, 33, 1861–1876.

Paoli, A., Siow, R., & Moro, T. (2025). Editorial: Spotlight on aging: Role of exercise and nutrition in healthy longevity. Frontiers in Aging, 6, 1698219.

Papadopoulou, S. K., Detopoulou, P., Voulgaridou, G., Tsoumana, D., Spanoudaki, M., Sadikou, F., Papadopoulou, V. G., Zidrou, C., Chatziprodromidou, I. P., Giaginis, C., & Kotsa, K. (2023). Mediterranean diet and sarcopenia features in apparently healthy adults over 65 years: A systematic review. Nutrients, 15(5), 1104.

Pedersen, B. K. (2019). Physical activity and muscle–brain crosstalk. Nature Reviews Endocrinology, 15(7), 383–392.

Pence, J., et al. (2025). Hydration strategies in older adults. Nutrients.

Peterson, M. D., Sen, A., & Gordon, P. M. (2011). Influence of resistance exercise on lean body mass in aging adults: A meta-analysis. Medicine & Science in Sports & Exercise, 43(2), 249–258.

Phillips, S. M. (2017). Nutritional supplements in support of resistance exercise to counter age-related sarcopenia. Advances in Nutrition, 8(2), 452–460.

Piovezan, R. D., Abucham, J., Dos Santos, R. V. T., et al. (2015). The impact of sleep on age-related sarcopenia: Possible connections and clinical implications. Ageing Research Reviews, 23(Pt B), 210–220.

Pourmotabbed, A., Ghaedi, E., Babaei, A., et al. (2020). Sleep duration and sarcopenia risk: A systematic review and dose-response meta-analysis. Sleep and Breathing, 24, 1267–1278.

Prinz, P. N., Scanlan, J. M., Vitaliano, P. P., et al. (1983). Plasma growth hormone during sleep in young and aged men. The Journal of Clinical Endocrinology & Metabolism, 56(2), 320–324.

Putra, C., Konow, N., Gage, M., York, C. G., & Mangano, K. M. (2021). Protein source and muscle health in older adults: A literature review. Nutrients, 13(3), 743.

Qi, P., Fu, S., et al. (2024). Effects of vitamin D supplementation on muscle strength in middle-aged and elderly individuals: A retrospective propensity score-matched study. Frontiers in Nutrition, 11, 1450265.

Qiu, Y., Fernández-García, B., Lehmann, H. I., et al. (2025). Exercise attenuates the hallmarks of aging: Novel perspectives. Journal of Sport and Health Science, 101108.

Rantanen, T., et al. (1999). Midlife hand grip strength as a predictor of old age disability. JAMA, 281(6), 558–560.

Reid-McCann, R. J., et al. (2025). Effect of plant versus animal protein on muscle mass, strength, physical performance, and sarcopenia: A systematic review and meta-analysis of randomized controlled trials. Nutrition Reviews.

Reid-McCann, R. J., et al. (2025). Effect of plant versus animal protein on muscle mass: Systematic review and meta-analysis. Nutrition Reviews.

Rich, A., Malliaras, P., Barton, C. J., et al. (2025). Treatment of proximal hamstring tendinopathy with education and exercise: A systematic review. Sports Medicine - Open, 11, 58.

Rolland, Y., Guyonnet, S., & Vellas, B. (2024). Therapeutic perspectives of pre-, pro-, and post-biotics in the treatment of sarcopenia. Nutrition Clinique et Métabolisme, 38(4), 307–313.

Rowe, G. C., & Arany, Z. (2014). Genetic models of mitochondrial dysfunction and ageing. Trends in Endocrinology & Metabolism, 25(10), 493–501.

Rubio-Arias, J. Á., Ávila-Gandía, V., López-Román, F. J., et al. (2019). Sleep quality and the prevalence of sarcopenia in older adults: A systematic review with meta-analysis. Journal of Clinical Medicine, 8(12), 2156.

Rueggeberg, R., Wrosch, C., Miller, G. E., et al. (2012). Sleep duration buffers diurnal cortisol increases in older adulthood. Psychoneuroendocrinology, 37(3), 382–390.

Ruiz-Valenzuela, R. E., Artacho, R., Ruiz-López, M. D., & Molina-Montes, E. (2025). Healthy dietary patterns and risk of sarcopenia in adults aged >50 years: A systematic review and meta-analysis considering EWGSOP1 and EWGSOP2 criteria. Nutrients, 17(17), 2764.

Saner, N. J., Lee, M. J. C., Pitchford, N. W., et al. (2020). The effect of sleep restriction, with or without high-intensity interval exercise, on myofibrillar protein synthesis in healthy young men. The Journal of Physiology, 598(8), 1523–1536.

Sathyakumar, S., Nair, A., & colleagues. (2025). Type 2 diabetes and sarcopenia. Journal of the Association of Physicians of India, 73(4), 11–16.

Schoenfeld, B. J., Grgic, J., Van Every, D. W., & Plotkin, D. L. (2021). Loading recommendations for muscle strength, hypertrophy, and local endurance: A re-examination of the repetition continuum. Sports, 9(2), 32.

Sharma, S., Bhadra, R., Selvam, S., et al. (2024). Vitamin B12 status and skeletal muscle function among elderly: A literature review and pilot study on the effect of oral vitamin B12 supplementation in improving muscle function. Aging Medicine, 7(4), 480–489.

Short, K. R., Bigelow, M. L., Kahl, J., Singh, R., Coenen-Schimke, J., Raghavakaimal, S., & Nair, K. S. (2005). Decline in skeletal muscle mitochondrial function with aging in humans. Proceedings of the National Academy of Sciences, 102(15), 5618–5623.

Silva, R., Pizato, N., da Mata, F., Figueiredo, A., Ito, M. K., & Pereira, M. G. (2018). Mediterranean diet and musculoskeletal-functional outcomes in community-dwelling older people: A systematic review and meta-analysis. Journal of Nutrition, Health and Aging, 22(6), 655–663.

Smeuninx, B., et al. (2020). Amount, source and pattern of dietary protein intake and muscle health. Frontiers in Nutrition.

Smeuninx, B., Greig, C. A., & Breen, L. (2020). Amount, source and pattern of dietary protein intake across the adult lifespan: A cross-sectional study. Frontiers in Nutrition, 7, 25.

Smith, B. E., Hendrick, P., Bateman, M., et al. (2025). Effectiveness of painful versus non-painful exercise on pain and function in chronic musculoskeletal pain: A systematic review and meta-analysis. Journal of Orthopaedic & Sports Physical Therapy, 55(3), 1–16.

Smith, G. I., et al. (2011). Omega-3 fatty acids augment the muscle protein anabolic response to hyperinsulinemia–hyperaminoacidemia in healthy young and middle-aged men and women. Clinical Science, 121(6), 267–278.

Soltanieh, S., Jayedi, A., Zargar, M. S., et al. (2022). Sleep duration and the risk of dietary and appetite outcomes: A systematic review and dose-response meta-analysis of randomized controlled trials. Advances in Nutrition, 13(4), 1174–1191.

Song, Q., Wang, Y., Jiang, H., Li, H., Cheng, C., Huang, L., & Cao, H. (2024). Changes in the gut microbiota of patients with sarcopenia: A meta-analysis. Frontiers in Nutrition, 11, 1429242.

Souza, A. C. R., Vasconcelos, A. R., Dias, D. D., Komoni, G., & Name, J. J. (2023). The integral role of magnesium in muscle integrity and aging: A comprehensive review. Nutrients, 15(24), 5127.

Therdyothin, A., et al. (2025). n-3 PUFA supplementation effects on muscle protein synthesis and whole-body protein synthesis: Systematic review and meta-analysis. Nutrition Reviews.

Tsigos, C., Kyrou, I., Kassi, E., & Chrousos, G. P. (2020). Stress: Endocrine physiology and pathophysiology. In K. R. Feingold, B. Anawalt, A. Boyce, et al. (Eds.), Endotext. MDText.com, Inc.

Van Cauter, E., & Copinschi, G. (1996). Physiology of growth hormone secretion during sleep. The Journal of Pediatrics, 128(5 Pt 2), S32–S37.

Van Cauter, E., & Plat, L. (2000). Interrelationships between sleep and the somatotropic axis. Sleep, 23(Suppl. 4), S109–S117.

Van Cauter, E., Leproult, R., & Plat, L. (2000). Age-related changes in slow wave sleep and REM sleep and relationship with growth hormone and cortisol levels in healthy men. JAMA, 284(7), 861–868.

Van Elswyk, M. E., McNeill, S. H., & Miller, M. J. (2022). Dietary patterns and the risk of sarcopenia: A systematic review and meta-analysis. Current Developments in Nutrition, 6(5), nzac036.

Volkert, D., et al. (2019). ESPEN guideline on clinical nutrition and hydration in geriatrics. Clinical Nutrition.

Volkert, D., et al. (2022). ESPEN practical guideline: Clinical nutrition and hydration in geriatrics. Clinical Nutrition, 41, 958–989.

Volpi, E., Nazemi, R., & Fujita, S. (2004). Muscle tissue changes with aging. Current Opinion in Clinical Nutrition and Metabolic Care, 7(4), 405–410.

Walston, J. D. (2012). Sarcopenia in older adults. Current Opinion in Rheumatology, 24(6), 623–627.

Wang, G., Hu, Y., Zhang, X., Liu, D., Wang, Y., & Li, Y. (2025). Gut microbiota in patients with sarcopenia: A systematic review and meta-analysis. Frontiers in Nutrition, 12, 1514696.

Wang, Q., Zhao, X., Wang, S., & Lu, S. (2025). Sarcopenia and immune-mediated inflammatory diseases: Evaluating causality and exploring therapeutic targets for sarcopenia through Mendelian randomization. International Immunopharmacology, 144, 113687.

Wei, S., et al. (2023). Sarcopenic obesity: Epidemiology, pathophysiology, and clinical implications. Frontiers in Endocrinology.

Westerståhl, M., Frändin, K., Ekelund, U., et al. (2025). Rise and fall of physical capacity in a general population. Scandinavian Journal of Medicine & Science in Sports, 35(1), e70072.

World Health Organization. (2024, June 26). Nearly 1.8 billion adults at risk of disease from not doing enough physical activity. World Health Organization.

Wright, V. J., Schwartzman, J. D., Itinoche, R., & Wittstein, J. (2024). The musculoskeletal syndrome of menopause. Climacteric, 27(5), 466–472.

Wu, W., Zhang, Y., Chen, X., et al. (2025). Dietary protein requirements of older adults with sarcopenia: A narrative review. Frontiers in Nutrition, 12, 1486482.

Xiao, Y., et al. (2025). Effects of acute caffeine intake on muscular power during resistance exercise: A systematic review and meta-analysis. Frontiers in Nutrition, 12, 1686283.

Xie, Z., Liu, Y., Wang, H., et al. (2025). A review of mitochondrial dysfunction in diabetic sarcopenia. Journal of International Medical Research, 53(5), 3000605251355996.

Xiong, A., et al. (2024). Effects of active vitamin D analogues on muscle strength and falls in elderly individuals: Meta-analysis. Frontiers in Endocrinology.

Xu, Y., Li, H., Zhang, H., Wang, J., & Chen, L. (2025). The gut-muscle axis: A comprehensive review of the interplay between gut microbiota and skeletal muscle. Frontiers in Nutrition, 12, 1520917.

Yan, R., Liu, H., Zhang, Q., et al. (2025). Optimal resistance training prescriptions to improve muscle-related outcomes in older adults with sarcopenia: A systematic review and meta-analysis. BMC Geriatrics, 25, 268.

Yang, W., Li, H., Zhou, X., Chen, Y., & Zhang, Q. (2025). Gut dysbiosis in primary sarcopenia: Potential mechanisms and therapeutic implications. Frontiers in Nutrition, 12, 1527374.

Yiallouris, A., Tsioutis, C., Agapidaki, E., et al. (2019). Adrenal aging and its implications on stress responsiveness in humans. Frontiers in Endocrinology, 10, 54.

Yu, B., Cheng, Y., Li, J., et al. (2024). Sarcopenic obesity is associated with cardiometabolic multimorbidity in middle-aged and older adults. Nutrition, Metabolism and Cardiovascular Diseases, 34(10), 2477–2485.

Yu, H., Wang, L., Chen, Y., et al. (2025). Effects of exercise intervention on falls and balance function in older adults: A systematic review and meta-analysis. Frontiers in Aging, 6, 1253680.

Zaromskyte, G., et al. (2021). Evaluating the leucine trigger hypothesis: A systematic review. Frontiers in Nutrition.

Zeng, Q., Zhao, L., Zhong, Q., An, Z., & Li, S. (2024). Changes in sarcopenia and incident cardiovascular disease in prospective cohorts. BMC Medicine, 22, 607.

Zhang, C., Cheng, Y., Li, Y., et al. (2024). Research progress on the correlation between estrogen and skeletal muscle mass in women. Frontiers in Endocrinology, 15, 1494972.

Zhang, X., Liu, Y., Chen, J., et al. (2025). Effects of statins on sarcopenia with focus on mechanistic insights and clinical applications. Frontiers in Pharmacology, 16, 1669591.

Zhang, Y., Li, H., Sun, P., et al. (2025). Critical pathogenesis of autoimmune-associated sarcopenia. Interactive Journal of Medical Research, 14, e64456.

Zhao, J., et al. (2024). Associations of serum vitamin B12 biomarkers with muscle mass/function. Frontiers in Endocrinology.

Zhao, R., Dong, Y., Zheng, Q., & Yao, J. (2025). Exercise and nutrition strategies for sarcopenia in older adults: Evidence from a network meta-analysis based on EWGSOP and AWGS criteria. Frontiers in Nutrition, 12, 1685014.

Zuo, X., Chen, Z., Li, J., et al. (2023). Sarcopenia and cardiovascular diseases: A systematic review. Clinical Cardiology, 46(6), 594–603.

Österdahl, M. F., Ní Lochlainn, M., Welch, C., Rymer, J., Ashworth, M., Whitney, J., Duncan, E. L., & Steves, C. J. (2025). Systematic review on the relationship between menopausal hormone replacement therapy, sarcopenia, and sarcopenia-related parameters. Maturitas, 199, 108609.

Reader Notes

Reader Notes

www.ingramcontent.com/pod-product-compliance
Lightning Source LLC
LaVergne TN
LVHW052036200926
848481LV00005B/1692
* 9 7 8 1 7 6 3 7 0 0 5 1 2 *